Herpes
PREVENTION & TREATMENT

by Donald A. Kullman, M.D.
and Joel Klass, M.D.

Copyright © 1983, Compact Books, Inc.

Published by
COMPACT BOOKS, INC.
P.O. Box 6263
Hollywood, Florida 33021

Copyright ©1983 by COMPACT BOOKS, INC.

All rights reserved. No part of this book may be reproduced in any form or by any means whatsoever without the prior written permission of the Publisher, excepting brief quotes used in connection with reviews written specifically for inclusion in a magazine or newspaper.

Library of Congress Cataloging in Publication Data

Kullman, Donald A., 1928-
  Herpes prevention & treatment.

  Includes index.
  1. Herpes simplex. I. Klass, Joel, 1942-
II. Title.
RC147.H6K84 1984   6.6.95'18   83-20888
ISBN 0-936320-14-1 (pbk.)

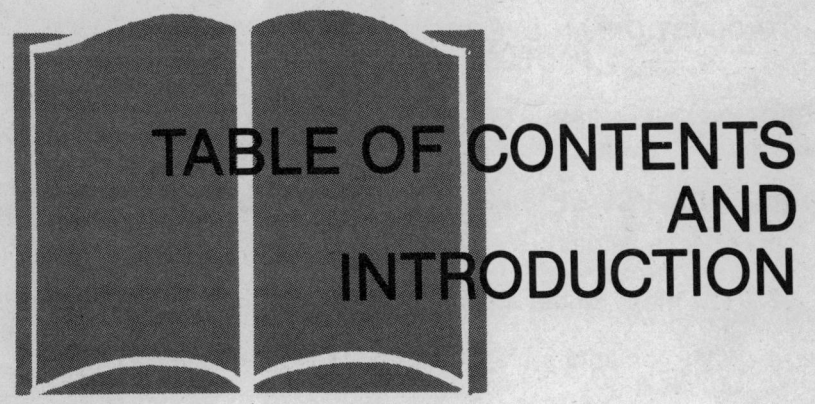

TABLE OF CONTENTS AND INTRODUCTION

Contents

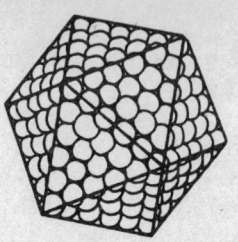

INTRODUCTION: AN OVERVIEW OF THE HERPES
PROBLEM............................ 8

SECTION ONE: HERPES QUESTIONS AND ANSWERS
By Donald A. Kullman, M.D.

PART I: DEFINING HERPES

1. What is herpes? 12
2. Can herpes recur?
3. How many kinds of herpes simplex viruses are there?
4. What conditions are caused by the herpes simplex viruses?
5. On what parts of the body are the lesions of herpes usually found?
6. Does each type of herpes simplex virus favor certain parts of the body? 14
7. Can HSV-1 sores be distinguished from HSV-2 sores?
8. Can herpes be cured? 15
9. Is herpes a new problem?
10. How widespread is oral herpes?
11. How widespread is genital herpes? 16

PART II: CONTRACTING HERPES

12. How is oral herpes usually acquired? 17
13. How does a person get genital herpes and/or lesions elsewhere on the body?
14. What does the term auto-inoculation mean? ....
15. How long after contact before a person develops herpes? 19
16. What is venereal disease?
17. Why is genital herpes considered to be a "sexually transmitted disease" (STD)?

18. Can oral herpes ever be considered a sexually transmitted disease? 20
19. If an individual has genital herpes, is it likely that he or she has another STD?
20. What does a herpes lesion look like?
21. What are the symptoms of genital herpes? 21
22. What other conditions can be confused with herpes eruptions? 22
23. Are canker sores the same as herpes? ....
24. How does herpes sometimes involve the rectum?
25. Do some people find they are unable to void after contracting herpes? 24
26. When are herpes infections most contagious? ......
27. Can a person have primary genital herpes without any symptoms?
28. Are silent recurrences common and are they contagious?
29. How long does an infection of genital herpes usually last? 26
30. Is it possible for a person to have a primary infection with one type of herpes simplex virus and then, years later, have another primary infection after exposure to another type or strain of virus?
31. Who suffers more from genital herpes, men or women? 27
32. Who suffers more after contracting genital herpes, the circumcised or the uncircumcised male?
33. Where, specifically, do the viruses hide between attacks, when they are dormant?
34. Does the virus affect the nerve along which it travels or the nerve center where it rests? 30
35. What causes herpes to recur?
36. What are prodromal symptoms?
37. Is it safe to have sexual relations during the prodromal period?
38. Does the presence of prodromal symptoms always herald a recurrence of the lesions? 31
39. What is the relationship between herpes recurrences and stress? 32
40. Does a severe primary infection imply more frequent and/or more severe recurrences? 33
41. How often do recurrent attacks of herpes occur?
42. Between attacks, can an infected person safely have

sex?
43. May two people with genital herpes safely have relations with each other when active lesions are present?
44. Can genital herpes be acquired by non-sexual means? 34
45. Can herpes be contracted from a toilet seat?
46. Can herpes be caught in a swimming pool or hot tub?
47. Can herpes be caught from a pet? 35
48. What is the most common clinical form of herpes?
49. How does herpes affect the eyes?
50. Does herpes sometimes infect the throat? 37
51. What is herpes eczema? 38
52. What is herpes meningitis?
53. What is herpes encephalitis? 39
54. How is herpes encephalitis treated?
55. Is ARA-A useful for genital herpes? 40
56. Are other forms of ARA-A helpful for herpes skin infections?
57. Does herpes sometimes involve the digestive tract?
58. Is there such a thing as chronic herpes simplex skin infections? 41
59. Does herpes sometimes infect the fingers?
60. Are medical personnel at risk for catching herpes infections? 42
61. Who usually contracts acute herpes of the mouth and gums?

PART III: DIAGNOSING HERPES

62. Should a person consult a physician if he or she suspects genital herpes? 43
63. How are herpes simplex viruses usually diagnosed?
64. Can a blood test be used to diagnose herpes? ......
65. What does a positive blood test mean?
66. Can a blood test be used to type the herpes simplex virus? 45
67. How can the exact type of herpes simplex virus (Type 1 or Type 2) be determined?
68. Is the typing of herpes easy to do?
69. Is it important to know what type of herpes virus is involved in a case of genital herpes?
70. Can a pap smear diagnose genital herpes? 46

PART IV: PREVENTION AND CONTROL OF HERPES

71. Is there any surefire way to prevent herpes? 47
72. If one is unwilling to follow the strict 1-2-3 program outlined previously, what constitutes a reasonable compromise program to protect an uninfected partner?
73. If one partner has genital herpes, what are the other partner's chances of contracting the disease, given repeated exposure? 48
74. What are the advantages of having only one sexual partner? 49
75. Will washing and urinating immediately following sexual relations also help to prevent herpes? 50
76. What can be done to reduce the incidence of recurrent attacks?
77. Do people sometimes become confused about who caught what from whom? 52
78. What is the role of sex education in schools in herpes prevention? 53

PART V: TREATMENTS FOR HERPES

79. What ineffective "cures" for herpes have been touted? 55
80. What is the placebo effect? 56
81. What is Acyclovir? 58
82. What other antiviral drugs are available? 59
83. What is Interferon?
84. What is the carbon dioxide laser treatment? 60
85. Can herpes symptoms be relieved with simple home remedies? 61
86. Is the development of a vaccine against herpes close at hand? 62

PART VI: HERPES AND PREGNANCY

87. May a pregnant woman engage in intercourse, without special considerations, if either she or her partner has or develops herpes? 63
88. What kind of herpes infection in a pregnant woman is potentially dangerous to the unborn child?
89. What may happen if a woman gets genital herpes for the first time late in pregnancy? 64
90. How great a special danger does herpes pose to the newborn?

91. Is the risk to the infant greater if the mother has a primary infection of herpes or if the mother is experiencing a recurrence of herpes at term? 66
92. What can be done to prevent congenital herpes? 68
93. What factors play a role in deciding whether to perform special lab tests and to consider doing a caesarean section at the time of delivery?
94. How many smears or cultures should be taken near term to determine if the virus is active and being shed?
95. Will delivery by caesarean section while the membranes are still intact guarantee the baby will not have herpes? 69
96. Can a newborn contract herpes postpartum even if its mother does not have genital herpes?

PART VII: HERPES AND CANCER

97. What is the relationship between herpes and cancer? 71

PART VIII: THE LIFE CYCLE OF THE HERPES VIRUS AND BODY DEFENSES

98. What is a virus? 73
99. What is the natural life cycle of the herpes virus? ... 76
100. How does the body protect itself from the onslaught of the herpes virus? 77

PART IX: THE SOCIOLOGICAL ASPECTS OF HERPES

101. What is the most important sociological step toward combatting herpes? 82
102. Has public thinking about herpes changed in the past few years?
103. Has the media caused fears about herpes to be blown out of proportion?
104. Has herpes affected attitudes toward sexual activity? 83
105. How has herpes affected attitudes toward the "one night stand"?
106. Do prostitutes have a high incidence of herpes infections?
107. Has herpes been affected by changes in birth control techniques?
108. Do many people overreact to herpes? 84

PART X: HERPES RESOURCES

109. Is there a resource that provides on-going information and counseling for individuals with herpes? 85

PART XI: AIDS

110. Does the homosexual community have a higher incidence of herpes, STD's in general, or a related problem? 86
111. What is Kaposi's Sarcoma?
112. Is Kaposi's sarcoma related to the AIDS? 87
113. What causes AIDS?
114. Does overwork cause the body's immune defense system to break down?
115. What are the symptoms of AIDS? 88
116. Is Kaposi's sarcoma the only type of malignancy associated with AIDS?
117. Is AIDS a new disorder?
118. How contagious is AIDS? 89
119. How is AIDS treated? 90
120. Is AIDS a fatal disorder? 91
121. How is AIDS diagnosed?
122. Is there a good side to AIDS?
123. How can individuals who need blood transfusions protect themselves against AIDS?
124. What is the single most important thing a male homosexual can do to avoid AIDS? 92
125. Should all contact with male homosexuals be avoided to protect against AIDS?
126. How important is hygiene in Aids prevention?
127. Where can an individual call for further information on AIDS?

PART XII: THE LEGAL ASPECTS OF HERPES

128. What are the lawsuits involving herpes that have received so much publicity recently all about? 93

SECTION TWO: THE PSYCHOLOGICAL DIMENSION
BY JOEL KLASS, M.D. 95

GLOSSARY 112
INDEX 120

The Herpes Problem: An Editorial Overview

Herpes is a subject on everyone's lips these days. What in the past was regarded as a simple cold sore arising from "innocent" causes, has now become one of the most prolific and persistent sexually transmitted diseases. Most individuals are unaware that herpes viruses cause not only the sexually-related lesions, but are also responsible for chickenpox, shingles and infectious mononucleosis ("mono"). Each of these diseases has been widespread for many years ... except for the herpes simplex which infects the genital area.

Even genital herpes is not new. In 1736, French physician Jean Astruc described genital herpes and in 1797, an English doctor named Bell mentioned the lesions of genital herpes in a treatise on venereal diseases. The disease was described in German medical literature by Fuchs in 1840, and in a dermatological text published in 1902, Crocker refers to genital herpes as "not uncommon".

What *is* new about genital herpes is the alarming rise in incidence over the past decade. The pool of those persons who harbor and thus are readily capable of spreading the disease enlarges by an estimated half-million new cases per year! Therefore, genital herpes now constitutes a major public health problem.

As recently as 15 years ago, genital herpes almost invariably was one of the strains known as herpes virus Type 2 (HSV-2). The common cold sore of the mouth area was just as invariably herpes simplex virus Type 1 (HSV-1). The sexual revolution brought this distinction to a screeching halt. It now is not at all uncommon for "above the waist" herpes to be an HSV-2 infection, and known cases of HSV-1 infections of the genital area are on the rise.

Herpes is often described as incurable, yet it is a self-limiting disease. Thus, while it never goes away, herpes at least does not worsen. Once infected by herpes, the virus will remain within the system permanently. Herpes alternates between periods of activity and periods of dormancy, both with unpredictable durations. Recurrences tend to occur progressively less often and become progressively less severe. The virus is relatively stable and ordinarily does not spread to other parts of the body, so the recurrent lesions are usually limited to the original site(s) of infestation.

Herpes lesions are painful, and the virus is a potential source of serious complications in pregnant women. Perhaps the saddest and most pitiful form of the disease is neonatal herpes, herpes of newborn infants. The virus also may be associated with the recent increase in the incidence of cervical cancer. Fortunately, most cases of both neonatal herpes and cervical cancer are preventable, simply through appropriate action. And the keys to this appropriate action are awareness and knowledge.

Since herpes cannot be cured, since the viral eruptions are of an unpredictable nature, and since the disease is now one of the most common known to humankind, awareness and knowledge may be the chief resources for coping successfully with the condition — whether an individual alone has herpes, his or her partner has it, or both have contracted the virus. And awareness and knowledge regarding herpes currently must assume added importance, in light of the lack of medical resources available to treat the disease.

Antiviral research and therapy is now in its infancy, similar to the status of antibiotics several decades ago. At that time, only a few basic antibiotics were available, and many diseases existed which were beyond their scope of application. Today there are a number of effective antibiotics, and many new drugs are now being tested as antiviral agents. So far, however, no "wonder drug" for herpes victims has been developed. None have proven capable of eradicating the virus from its haven of safety when dormant. There are several drugs currently available (e.g., acyclovir) which are effective in reducing the severity of herpes, but only of the initial attack. And in most cases, results are far from dramatic.

Antiviral medications have been developed and used successfully in cases of herpes of the eyes, currently the most common cause of infectious blindness in the United States. There also exist medications that have reduced substantially the fatality rate of herpes (of the brain — herpes encephalitis). Thus, it appears that viral research — along with cancer research, for in many respects the two are closely related — is coming of age. There is every reason to believe that the future holds hope and promise. Until research is more fruitful, however, only the symptoms of herpes can be treated, and only with varying degrees of success.

Perhaps even more taxing than the physical effects of herpes are the associated emotional difficulties for sufferers. The psychological trauma of contracting herpes can be devastating. Marriages and meaningful relationships have been destroyed since one or both partners may be unwilling or unable to make the required life adjustments the disease demands. In marital, romantic and social relationships, knowledge and awareness must provide the means for making possible the necessary adaptations to the realities of herpes.

This publication addresses the subject herpes in the most direct way: the promotion of knowledge and awareness. Like the unpredictability of the viral course itself, herpes can affect the life of each individual differently. Therefore, sufferers must formulate their own effective, successful perspective on the disease and the effects on their individual lives. It is the authors' intention that this publication will provide readers with the knowledge and awareness needed to do so.

DONALD A. KULLMAN, M.D.

The authors and editor gratefully acknowledge the generous resources made available to them from the Centers for Disease Control, Atlanta, Georgia.

The purpose of this publication is to describe the physical and emotional aspects of herpes virus infections. In no way is it intended to supplant or displace competent treatment, supervision and management of herpes infections by qualified physicians. Indeed, it is designed to support and enhance the cooperative effort which should exist between doctor and patient. Better informed individuals are more likely to avoid contracting the disease. For those individuals who already have herpes, the better informed they are about the disease, the more effective will be the medical treatment received from the physician, and the chances are reduced for spreading herpes to other parts of the body or to other persons.

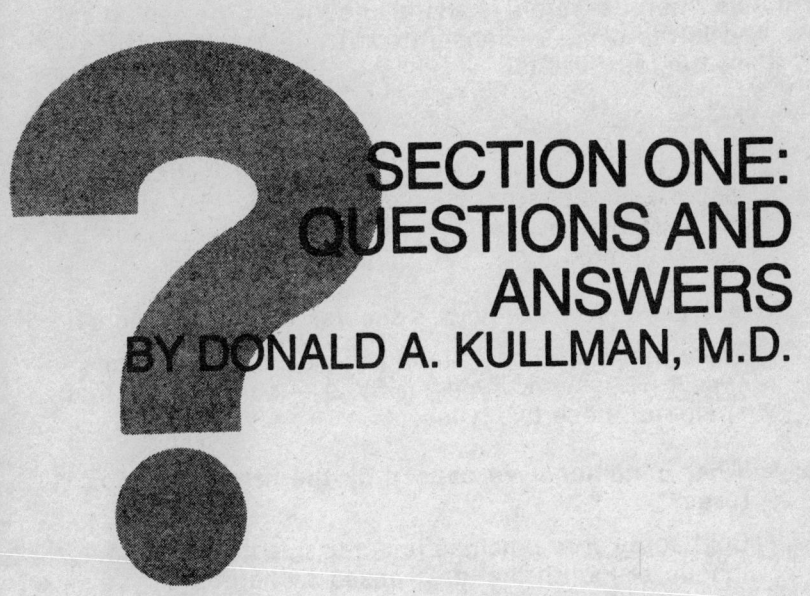

SECTION ONE: QUESTIONS AND ANSWERS
BY DONALD A. KULLMAN, M.D.

PART I:
Defining Herpes

1. What is herpes?

"Herpes" is the common term for an infection caused by the herpes simplex viruses. As generally used by the public, "herpes" refers to a viral infection of the genital area which is sexually transmitted. It is a painful and highly contagious disease.

2. Can herpes recur?

Once a person experiences an initial infection, he remains a carrier of the disease permanently. The virus may then alternate between states of dormancy and states of recurrent infection.

3. How many kinds of herpes simplex viruses are there?

There are two closely related herpes simplex viruses — Type 1 (HSV-1) and Type 2 (HSV-2) — but there are many strains of these two types.

4. What conditions are caused by the herpes simplex viruses?

Cold sores or oral herpes refers to infections of the lips, tongue or mouth that are caused by herpes simplex viruses. Ocular herpes occurs when herpes simplex virus infects the eyes. Herpes encephalitis is a serious, but infrequent, herpes simplex infection of the brain and spinal cord. Newborn babies may develop a severe form of herpes infection if born through an infected birth canal or infected soon after birth.

5. On what parts of the body are the lesions of herpes usually found?

The overwhelming majority of all herpes cases involves the mouth, lips, genital area, eyes and skin.

The usual areas infected by genital herpes are the external genitals. In men, these are the glans, or head, of the penis, the foreskin of and shaft of the penis and the area about the rectum (Fig. 1). In women, these are the labia majora and labia minora, foreskin of the clitoris, the fourchette — the area between the vagina and the rectum — and the rectum (Fig. 2). Internally, the urethra (the channel which carries urine from the bladder) in both man and woman and the vagina and cervix (the neck of the womb) of a woman are not uncommon sites of infestation. The thighs and buttocks are also frequent sites for the herpes sores.

Recurrent genital infections in females are generally external and not intravaginal. This change in location is analogous to oral herpes lesions which are within the mouth with primary infections and generally on the lips with recurrent attacks.

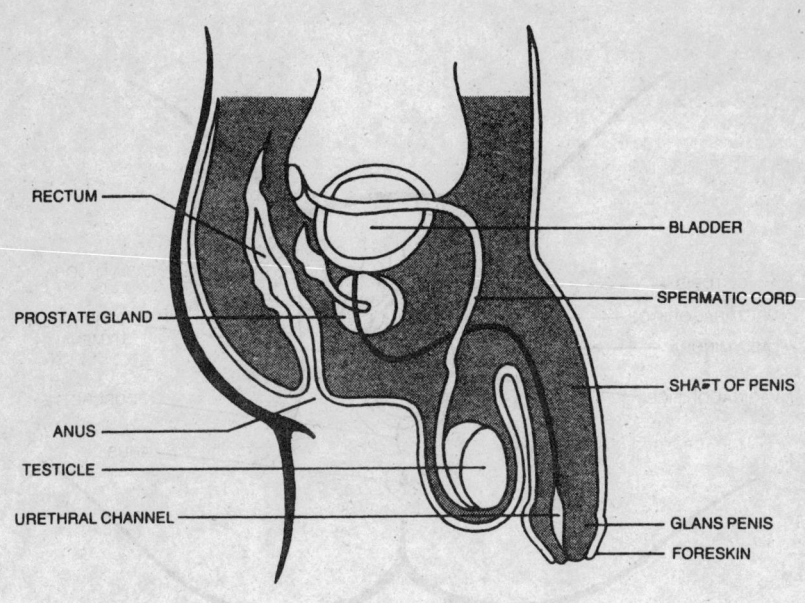

Fig. 1 – Male Genitals

6. Does each type of herpes simplex virus favor certain parts of the body?

For many years, HSV-1 was seldom found below the waist while HSV-2 was seldom found above it. With the change in sexual practices over the past decade or two, the classical description of the two viral types has altered. Due particularly to the rise in oral-genital sex, now about 20 to 25 percent of all genital herpes are HSV-1 infections. Due to the same rise in oral-genital sex, HSV-2 infections are becoming increasingly frequent to the area about the mouth.

7. Can HSV-1 sores be distinguished from HSV-2 sores?

From general appearances, lesions caused by either of the two strains of herpes viruses can not be told apart. They can be differentiated only by specific laboratory studies.

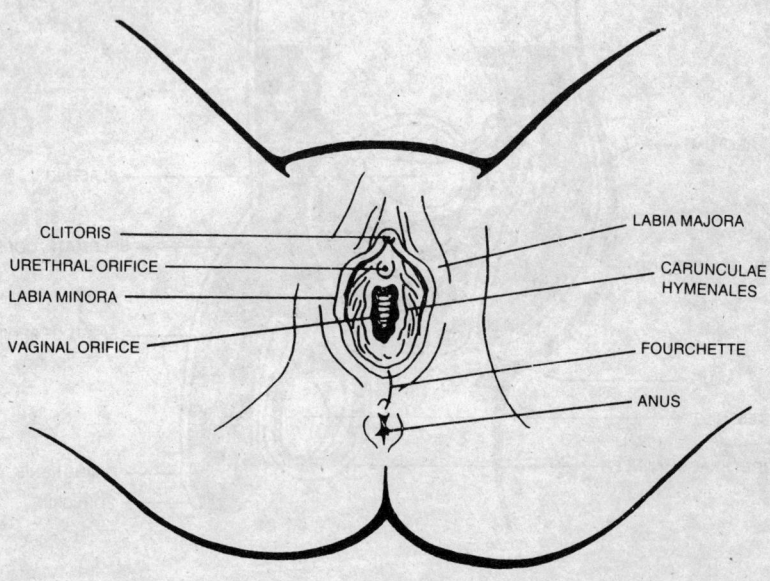

Fig. 2 – Female Genitals

8. Can herpes be cured?

No, technically herpes is an incurable affliction. But, contrary to popular belief, herpes is not serious, nor is it fatal. Herpes does not lead to progressive degeneration of the body, nor to serious consequences — even when untreated. In fact, herpes tends to lessen with each recurrence. Like the common cold, people recover from herpes despite the fact that there is no known cure. Once herpes is contracted, however, the virus stays in the body for life. Herpes does not kill, but it cannot be killed*

> *Note:* Recently, an experimental treatment using focused laser beams was successful with primary cases of herpes. At present, this treatment method is very expensive and not widely available. It is still being researched and has yet to be a proven cure for herpes.

9. Is herpes a new problem?

Herpes has probably existed for a long time: symptoms were noted more than 2,000 years ago. In ancient Rome, the Emperor Tiberius banned kissing in order to prevent the spread of the disease.

The first actual recorded incidence of herpes involving the genital tract was made by Jean Astruc in 1736. While Astruc described the condition, he did not name it. In 1814 Thomas Batemen applied the term "herpes" to genital lesions. In the 1880's, pathologists recognized the changes which occur within the body's cells as a result of herpes. By this time, genital herpes had become fairly common in VD clinics.

10. How widespread is oral herpes?

Herpes of the mouth is far more common than most people imagine. Herpes frequently occurs without symptoms. Until the 1920's oral infection during childhood was almost 100%. Currently, as a result of public health measures, this figure has been reduced to approximately 60%. This means that 120,000,000 Americans have had contact with HSV-1, and more than half have developed the characteristic cold sores and mouth blisters.

Generally, a first attack of herpes (one which does have symptoms) produces lesions in the mouth. Cold sores on the lips are more common in later attacks. And the cold sores from fever or sunburn are forms of herpes, usually short-lived but a potential source of future problems.

11. How widespread is genital herpes?

Herpes defies the old saying, "nothing is forever". Since herpes is a disease without a cure, health departments do not consider the virus as "reportable". Therefore, the medical community is not required to report herpes cases, so estimates on prevalency are only "guestimates" and tend to be on the low side.

The best available estimate for the prevalence of herpes is 20,000,000 cases, or around ten percent of the United States population. About 500,000 new cases of genital herpes develop each year. With such a growth rate, health departments may eventually mandate some form of reporting for herpes, especially if medical advances in herpes treatment occur.

Having reached what by any standards would be considered epidemic proportions, the subject of herpes is generating widespread interest and concern among healthcare professionals and the general public.

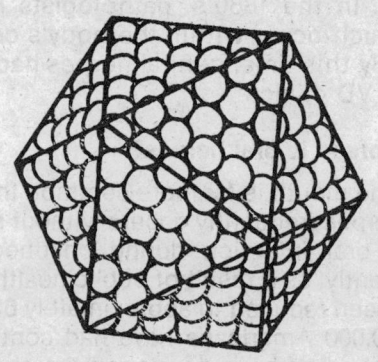

PART II:
Contracting Herpes

12. **How is oral herpes usually acquired?**

    Most primary cases of oral herpes are seen in young children. Children get this form of herpes from the active cold sores of adults and older children who care for or play with the youngsters. Direct contact, often momentary, is all that is necessary to pass the virus. Most cases of oral herpes in adults are believed to be reactivations of latent infections that were acquired in childhood. However, new primary cases of oral herpes in adults undoubtedly also occur.

13. **How does a person get genital herpes and/or lesions elsewhere on the body?**

    Herpes has been nicknamed the "virus of love". Intimate body contact is usually required in order to spread the virus from an infected to an uninfected person. To get herpes, an active herpes lesion must have contact with a susceptible skin or mucous membrane area.

    Actually, any part of the body is susceptible to being infected by the herpes virus. The mucous membranes are vulnerable as they are, while the type of abrasion required for the virus to penetrate the intact skin is ever so minor (Fig. 3). A lesion can develop on any part of the body the virus succeeds in infecting.

    Herpes can also be spread manually. For instance, if you touched a person's herpes lesion and then rubbed your eye with the same finger, your eye could become infected.

    Saliva can contain active herpes virus with oral herpes, and semen or vaginal secretions may contain the active virus in cases of genital herpes. Only the imagination can limit the routes possible for the herpes virus during sexual activity: oral-to-oral, genital-to-genital, oral-to-genital, genital-to-oral, and genital-rectal. Once infected, an area is capable of infecting in turn.

    Oral-genital contact accounts for much of the increase in

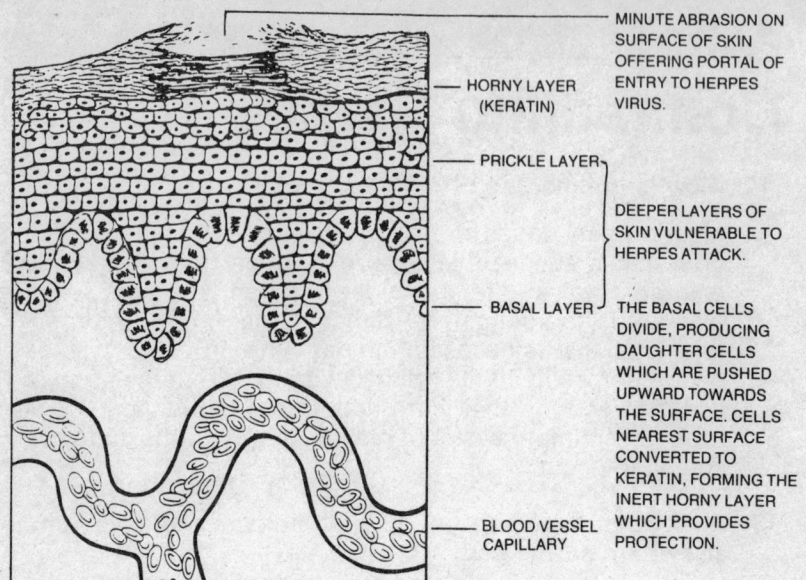

Fig. 3 – Schematic Drawing of Skin

genital herpes. HSV-1 is nearly universal. Kissing is its most common transmitter. The membranes of the genital area are especially susceptible to infection from the herpes virus. These factors in conjunction mean one person's cold sore can become another person's genital herpes. Then, once infected with genital herpes, genital herpes is spread further by the more common genital-to-genital contact.

14. What does the term auto-inoculation mean?

Auto-inoculation or, as it is also called, self-inoculation means to infect yourself by transporting a contagious substance (in this case, the herpes virus) from one, infected, portion of your body to another, uninfected portion. The most common vehicle of auto-inoculation is the hand, although this need not be the case every time. A fairly common cause of herpes of the eyes is the moistening of contact lenses with contaminated saliva.

A female with herpes of the lip, may touch her lip, and then insert a tampon or diaphragm without washing her hands, thus spreading the virus to the genital area.

Herpes of the fingers, too, can develop through auto-inoculation, the source again being contaminated saliva or contact with a genital lesion. These are just several very obvious yet all-too-frequently overlooked modes of auto-inoculation. Auto-inoculation is more likely to occur with a primary infection than with a recurrent one.

15. How long after contact before a person develops herpes?

The time that elapses between the entrance of the virus into the body following exposure to the virus, and the onset of symptoms, is called the incubation period. The incubation period of the herpes virus can vary greatly from individual to individual, symptoms appearing as soon as two days following infection and as late as 20 days following exposure to the virus. The average incubation period is about six days.

16. What is venereal disease?

The term venereal disease, or as it is abbreviated VD, refers to any disease transmitted from one person to another by any combination of genital contact; i.e. genital to genital, oral to genital, or hand to genital. Recently both venereal disease and VD have been supplanted by the more accurate and more socially acceptable euphemism — sexually transmitted disease (STD).

17. Why is genital herpes considered to be a "sexually transmitted disease" (STD)?

For genital herpes to occur for the first time, intimate contact with a partner who has active herpes is usually necessary. In the overwhelming majority of cases, therefore, genital herpes is sexually transmitted. Such intimate contact need not be limited to sexual intercourse. Genital herpes may be contracted through mutual masturbation if one of the participants fingers are contaminated with infected secretions and may be contracted through oral-genital sexual activity if the sexual partner has herpes of the lip. The term genital herpes refers to the site of infection, not to the strain of the infecting virus nor the mode of infection.

The sole criterion for genital herpes is a herpes infection

of the genital area. It makes no difference whether the infecting strain is the Type 1 herpes simplex virus or the Type 2 herpes simplex virus.

18. Can oral herpes ever be considered a sexually transmitted disease?

Yes, but only if it is acquired through oral-genital sex. Herpes simplex virus from active genital sores may be spread to the mouth area of the partner under these circumstances.

19. If an individual has genital herpes, is it likely that he or she has another STD?

STD's are widespread, and are often associated with one another. An individual who has contracted genital herpes is at risk for having contracted another STD, so proper medical management of the herpes patient dictates an active search for a concurrent STD. Some STD's such as syphilis or gonorrhea, have a more serious potential than does herpes for causing long range complications. The symptoms of one STD can mask symptoms of another. Since the symptoms of herpes are often so pronounced, they can hide those of another, more serious STD. Thus, if an individual has herpes, it is imperative to insure that any other STD's are diagnosed and treated as well.

One clinical study reported three out of every ten women coming to the clinic for birth control information and a routine examination had gonorrhea yet were unaware of the presence of the condition. That is 30%. While so high a figure in part can be attributed to the poor socio/economic conditions of these clinic patients, and thus 30% would certainly not be representative of the entire country, the point nevertheless is well-taken that sexually transmitted diseases often elude discovery.

20. What does a herpes lesion look like?

The first sign of herpes is a red dot or crops of bumps at the site of infection. This develops into a blister which is filled with clear fluid which gradually becomes thick and yellow. After a day or two, the blisters become ulcerated, then crusty and scab-like. Usually, there is more than one lesion in the area, and sometimes, they merge into a single, larger lesion. Gradually the scabs fall off as the lesions heal over and disappear without scarring.

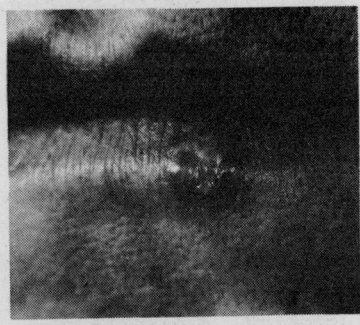

Herpes simplex lesion of lower lip. Second day after onset.

21. What are the symptoms of genital herpes?

Often the earliest symptoms of genital herpes is burning or itching at the site of infection. This unpleasant sensation is followed by the painful herpes lesions: the blisters, filled with fluid.

During the active phase of the lesions, systemic flu-like symptoms are often present, and sometimes are quite severe during initial infections. These symptoms include fever, loss of appetite, general malaise and of course, local pain and swelling in the genital area. When the lesions involve the urethra — the channel which leads from the bladder to the exterior — the resultant inflammation causes pain or burning upon urination. Similarly, when rectal or perianal lesions are present, there is pain with bowel movements. Some vaginal discharge is common in the female, and intercourse can be painful when vaginal lesions are present. Surprisingly, in most women, cervical lesions *alone* usually are not painful at all. This is because the cervix is a rather insensitive structure, lacking pain receptors.

Although there are no absolute rules, in cases of genital herpes (particularly in females) there is often a generalized pelvic ache and painful swellings along the groin.

These are the swollen inguinal lymph nodes. The symptoms of a primary attack tend to be far more pronounced and prominent than those of recurrent attacks. Some persons with apparently mild infections, however, suffer much while others, with what appear to be extensive lesions, seem to have only minimal symptoms, and occasionally do not suffer at all. Very rarely, a primary herpes infection of the genital tract can be severe enough to warrant hospitalization.

22. **What other conditions can be confused with herpes eruptions?**

The medical history may be as important as the physical examination when making the diagnosis of herpes. Previous episodes of lesions, or a history of a partner known to have active genital herpes or cold sores can provide important clues. When the presenting lesions display the classical picture: blisters with reddened borders and fluid-filled centers which rupture and leave grey ulcerations, accurate diagnosis is not likely to be a problem. It should be noted, however, that the blisters easily rupture and are not commonly seen in the female with genital herpes. Also, there are many cases which are atypical and do not resemble the textbook description of herpes. And, there are other dermatological conditions which superficially — that is, to the eye — may resemble the usual presenting picture of herpes.

Small boils (medically called folliculitis), infections caused by staph bacteria, at the base of hair follicles; scabies and other minor skin irritations; chancroid, a less common bacterial sexually transmitted disease; each of these as well as syphilis, the so-called "great imitator disease" can be and has been confused with herpes. Physicians routinely test the blood for syphilis when first treating a patient with herpes; and if the test is negative another blood test will be made one or two months later as well, for the organisms which cause syphilis may require that much time to cause the body to show a positive reaction in the blood.*

*Physicians should be aware that the FTA (Fluorescent Treponema Antibody Absorption test) is often misleading in the presence of genital herpes. False positive tests are common. Dark field examination of the lesions for the spirochetes that cause syphilis is necessary if a misdiagnosis is to be avoided.

23. Are canker sores the same as herpes?

Though often confused with one another, canker sores and herpes are unrelated. Medically called aphthous ulcers, the cause of canker sores is unknown; no infectious organisms can be cultured from them. Their coloring is greyish-white, surrounded by a bright red border. Canker sores usually occur inside the lips, inside the cheeks or at the base of the gums, yet can occur almost anywhere within the mouth. A sore will last from ten days to two weeks. Like herpes, recurrent attacks can be prompted by emotional or physical stress, strenuous physical activity or diet. Unlike herpes, canker sores are not contagious.

24. How does herpes sometimes involve the rectum?

Genital herpes may be spread to the anal area by contact from a finger just previously in contact with an infected lesion in the genital area or elsewhere on the body. The rise in the practice of anal intercourse accounts for the rising rate in cases of herpes involving the rectum. Herpes, then, has a perfect respect for "gay rights", and truly is an "equal opportunity infector". However, contrary to much opinion, anal intercourse is not the exclusive province of homosexual males.

When rectal pain, difficulty in urinating, pain in the thighs or in the buttocks and strange sensations on or beneath the skin exist, rectal herpes is likely.

About two-thirds of those who have rectal herpes will have vesicles or ulcers either in the rectal canal or in the perianal area, and about the same percentage also will exhibit swelling in the groin of the inguinal lymph nodes.

Bowel movements can cause severe pain, as the stool passes over the open, raw ulcerations within the rectum. In such instances, stool softeners are prescribed to reduce this pain. Keeping the rectal area dry and clean limits the further spread of the virus.

Any male presenting himself to a physcan for treatment of a proctitis — an inflamation of the mucous membranes of the rectum — should have a viral culture performed to rule out herpes. A significant percentage of such cultures will prove to be positive.

Rectal herpes has been mistakenly diagnosed as rectal gonorrhea, although as physicians have become better acquainted with this form of herpes such confusion has been substantially less. To compound matters, herpes and rectal gonorrhea are not mutually exclusive. In fact, one study revealed that in one-fourth of the cases of rectal herpes gonorrhea or syphilis coexisted.

25. Do some people find they are unable to void after contracting herpes?

Yes. Urinary retention is a common complication in females with genital herpes and males with rectal herpes. When the herpes lesions affect the urethra, voiding is likely to be difficult and painful. These symptoms, often associated with fever, tend to cause the individual to reduce fluid intake. The urine then becomes more concentrated. When there is poor emptying of the bladder and concentrated urine, the stage is set for bacterial infection.

It is important for those who develop this complication to force themselves to drink a lot of fluids — which will dilute the urine and the concentration of uric acid in the urine. Uric acid is the main chemical responsible for the burning and pain. One way to reduce the discomfort of voiding is to sit in a tub of warm water up to the hips, the so-called "sitz bath", and then void while in the tub. Another way is to pour warm water over the external vaginal lips and yet another method is to apply warm compresses to the area.

In extreme cases, when urinating causes severe pain, the individual may require a catheter to be inserted into the bladder, being left in place until the lesions and the pain from them subside.

Like herpes attacks in general, recurrent attacks of the urinary tract tend to be milder, heal more rapidly and recur less frequently. Some pain and perhaps a mild burning may be present in a recurrent attack, yet chills and fever tend to be rare.

26. When are herpes infections most contagious?

Herpes is most contagious when the sores are present and continues to be highly contagious until the sores are healed and the scabs have cleared up.

27. Can a person have primary genital herpes without any symptoms?

Yes, it is possible to be infected without developing visible lesions, but this is not common. Such infections occur without symptoms, or the symptoms are so mild that they are not detected. In retrospect, many persons who claim to have been asymptomatic, can actually recall some sort of sores which were dismissed as pimples, ingrown hairs, etc.

28. Are silent recurrences common and are they contagious?

Yes and yes. Recurrent episodes often are mild. The minimal blistering may not be noticed or the entire episode may be completely asymptomatic. Although the exact extent of silent viral shedding is unknown, current estimates range from two percent to twenty percent of women with herpes, with most authorities leaning toward the conservative figure.* Men, also, may have silent recurrences such as those which might occur in the mucous membrane of the urethral channel in the penis. While no sores would be present, the semen will contain virus particles. The percentage of males with genital herpes who exhibit silent shedding is probably less than one percent. Even apparently healed skin lesions can sometimes shed virus, although this is quite uncommon. Whether silent or loud, invisible or blatantly obvious, all herpes recurrences are to be considered highly contagious.

*The amount of virus shed in the absence of active lesions is considerably less than when lesions are present, consequently the infectivity of the silent shedder is not nearly as great as the individual with visible lesions.

29. How long does an infection of genital herpes usually last?

On the average, an initial infection will last about two to three weeks, and the healing phase for another ten or eleven days. Because of the frequent involvement of the cervix and the larger surface area of the mucous membranes of the vagina exposed to the virus, women generally have more prolonged and more severe infections than men.

On the average again, a later, recurrent attack will last about five days. Due emphasis should be placed on the words "average" and "about", rather than on "three weeks" and "five days". The precise period an actual infection will last, whether initial or recurrent, can and very often does vary significantly from individual to individual.

The length and severity of an individual bout of herpes is determined by the location of the infections, and quantity of viral particles invading the host, the virulence of the particular strain of virus and the efficiency of the body's immune defense system. Those who have never had any herpes simplex infections, (cold sores, fever blisters, etc.) tend to have more severe infections because their immune defense systems are unprepared to fight the herpes virus.

30. Is it possible for a person to have a primary infection with one type of herpes simplex virus and then, years later, have another primary infection after exposure to another type or strain of virus?

Yes. For example, during childhood, a girl may get herpes Type 1 cold sores. As a young adult, this same person may be exposed to herpes Type 2 in the genital area and have a new primary infection with the Type 2 virus. That same person may later be exposed to a different strain of Type 2 virus and develop another primary infection.

31. Who suffers more from genital herpes, men or women?

While generally an impartial and democratic virus, when it comes to physical suffering herpes has a touch of male chauvinism to it. Women often develop lesions in areas that are warm and moist. Such blisters break easily, spread easily and are a source of considerable pain. Men undoubtedly fare better than do women. The average duration of an initial episode is about two weeks in men while it not uncommonly lasts about a week longer in women. Similarly, recurrent attacks are briefer in duration in men than they are in women. In both initial and recurrent episodes, the pain and intensity of an attack is less in men and the lesions are less likely in men to interfere with intercourse, although one should not engage in intercourse during an active attack of herpes, initial or recurrent.

32. Who suffers more after contracting genital herpes, the circumcised or the uncircumcised male?

The membranous tissue lining the foreskin of the uncircumcised male tends to remain moist. Because of this, uncircumcised males more frequently have prolonged infections and run a greater chance of the disease spreading to other sites than do circumcised males. In this country, the vast majority of males are circumcised, routinely and shortly after birth. The relative benefits circumcision offers if genital herpes is contracted must be regarded as a further recommendation for the procedure.

33. Where specifically do the viruses hide between attacks, when they are domant?

Between attacks the virus retreats into the nerve ganglion* nearest to the site of infection. Each area of the body is connected with, and monitored by, one or more nerve fibers, depending upon the location and size of the area in question.

Each nerve fiber in the body is a single cell, and nerve cells are the longest cells in the body, some measuring up to three feet in length in a tall person. Each sensory nerve cell extends from the area of the body it serves, which is the point where the nerve fiber ends in the skin or mucous membrane, to the spinal cord ganglion, which is where the nucleus of the nerve cells is located. A ganglion is a cluster or aggregate of nerve cells. The spinal ganglia are the central headquarters for the many nerve fibers which transmit sensory impulses, or feelings, from the skin or mucous membranes to the brain. The body's nervous system is not unlike a telephone switchboard: each individual telephone set (the receptors in the skin) stretching out from a central network (the spinal ganglia).

When a herpes outbreak abates, the virus is said to be in a dormant stage, similar to hibernation.

The sensory nerves supplying the oral cavity — the usual site of HSV-1 infestation — have their ganglia near the base of the brain in a pair of nerve clusters called the trigeminal ganglia. The trigeminal ganglia serve the mouth, lips, eyes and face (Fig. 4).

The sensory nerves supplying the genital area — the usual site of HSV-2 infestation — are rooted in the sacral ganglia, at the lower portion of the spinal cord. As a herpes attack of the mouth or lips subsides, the viruses retreat to the trigeminal ganglia, where they become dormant. As a herpes infestation of the genital area subsides, the viruses retreat to the sacral ganglia where they too become dormant.

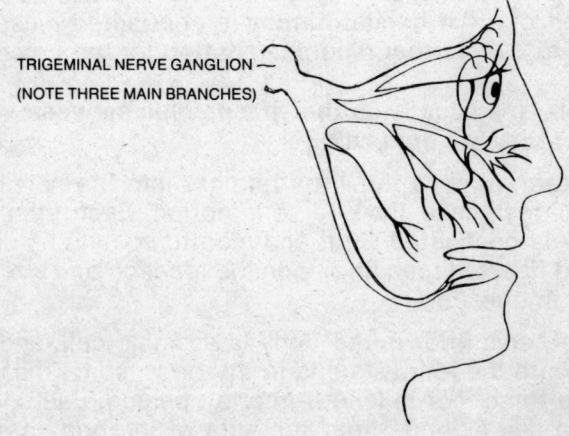

TRIGEMINAL NERVE GANGLION
(NOTE THREE MAIN BRANCHES)

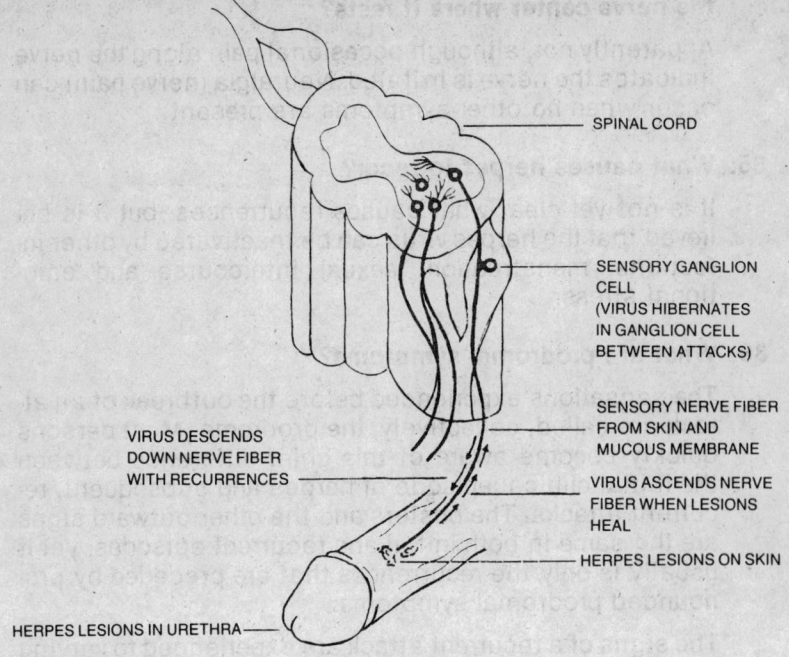

Fig. 5 – Spine/Penis Showing Path of Herpes Virus

When reactivation of the virus occurs, the virus reverses its former path, and this time travels from the ganglion of the nerve, along the fiber to the point where the nerve fiber ends: on the body's surface or mucous membrane at the site of the original lesion. There the virus once again replicates, forming another blister, which will last until the infection is once more controlled by the body's immune defense system and the virus retraces its steps back to the nerve ganglion and becomes dormant once more (Fig. 5).

As can be seen, unless herpes is spread physically and externally from one part of the body to another, it usually is a very localized virus, always recurring in precisely the same specific locations on the body's surface.

*Ganglion is singular; ganglia plural.

34. Does the virus affect the nerve along which it travels or the nerve center where it rests?

Apparently not, although occasional pain along the nerve indicates the nerve is irritated. Neuralgia (nerve pain) can occur when no other symptoms are present.

35. What causes herpes to recur?

It is not yet clear what causes recurrences, but it is believed that the herpes virus can be reactivated by other infections, menstruation, sexual intercourse and emotional stress.

36. What are prodromal symptoms?

The sensations experienced before the outbreak of an attack are called, collectively, the prodrome. Most persons quickly become aware of this chief difference between the initial clinical episode of herpes and subsequent, recurrent attacks. The blisters and the other outward signs are the same in both initial and recurrent episodes, yet it usually is only the recurrences that are preceded by pronounced prodromal symptoms.

The signs of a recurrent attack are experienced to varying degrees by different individuals. Some have no warning signs; about a third have painless symptoms, while most herpes victims experience mild to moderate discomfort and any of the following: crawling feelings, heat sensations, throbbing, tingling, burning, itching, "pins and needles", fatigue, and general malaise. Neuralgia, or pain along infected nerves, can often radiate from the buttocks to the knees and the skin may become sensitive. Myalgia, or pain in the muscles in the area of the infected nerves, is also common.

37. Is it safe to have sexual relations during the prodromal period?

Prodromal symptoms are warning signs that a recurrent attack is imminent, and usually will begin several hours to several days following the onset of symptoms. It has been suggested that this 24 to 48 hour prodromal period corresponds to the length of time it takes the virus to make the trip from the nerve ganglion, along the nerve fiber to the nerve ending in the skin or mucous membrane. Even though lesions may not be visibly apparent during the prodromal stage, the virus nonetheless has the capacity to be shed once it reaches its goal. Partners should still take precautions even though actual lesions may not have been seen.

38. Does the presence of prodromal symptoms always herald a recurrence of the lesions?

Not always. Mild prodromal symptoms may occur without being followed by a full-blown eruption of lesions, just as a few dark clouds may gather without a thunderstorm developing.

Usually, when the virus becomes roused from its dormant state, it begins its journey from the nerve ganglion toward the site of the original lesion. During this journey, the prodromal symptoms are experienced. Also during this journey, the body's immune defense system is alerted and can contain the virus and force it to retreat. Thus the virus does not reach its objective: the skin cells or the cells of the mucous membrane where it planned to replicate and erupt into a lesion and the recurrence is aborted.

As time passes, the body becomes increasingly adept at manufacturing the specific antibodies effective against the virus. However, because the herpes virus spreads from cell to cell without entering the blood or tissue space, antibodies are ineffective in preventing recurrences. This explains how herpes infections recur despite high antibody titers against the virus in the blood. It is the cell-mediated component of the immunological system which plays the significant role in containing recurrent infections. With increasing experience the defensive cells become more expert at recognizing and successfully attacking the virus. This is why recurrences tend to decrease in severity, frequency and duration: the body does a better job fighting the virus when it reattacks.

Eating a nutritious and balanced diet and being in good physical health helps the body's immune defense system operate at maximum efficiency.

39. What is the relationship between herpes recurrences and stress?

One's mental state has a powerful effect upon the workings of the body's natural defenses. Stress and worry adversely alter the chemistry of the body, and can interfere with the performance of the defense system. A "calm, cool and collected" mind enhances the body's functioning, including that of the immune defense system. Next to sexual activity itself, stress is the most frequent triggering mechanism of recurrent infections.

Stress makes recurrences worse, whether or not it has triggered a particular recurrence. Stress management techniques can be effective in decreasing both the frequency and severity of recurrences. Stress management techniques are of two sorts. One is avoiding situations which promote stress and changing the individual behavioral patterns one has which lead to stress. The other is learning to deal with stress better as it occurs.

When such techniques are utilized when the prodromal symptoms are first noticed, recurrences can be prevented from proceeding further than that initial stage of warning. In other words, attacks can be prevented *with* psychological control which, *without* psychological control, would otherwise progress fully to the development of active lesions.

This form of stress management, while the preferable of the two forms, is the more difficult to learn.*

However, the relief it can provide and the suffering it can prevent make it well worth an attempt. Even moderate success at learning this form of stress management, while perhaps not likely to enable a recurrent attack to be aborted completely, can render recurrent attacks far more tolerable and briefer than they otherwise would be.

>*The spectrum of stress management techniques includes biofeedback, the same principles one learns in natural childbirth instruction, certain disciplines of yoga, Benson's Relaxation Response, TM, and other forms of meditation.

40. Does a severe primary infection imply more frequent and/or more severe recurrences?

Fortunately not. In fact there often seems to be an inverse correlation between the severity and/or frequency of recurrent attacks. It must be borne in mind, however, that all subsequent attacks are not necessarily recurrent attacks; they may be reinfections or they may be new infections of previously uninfected areas.

41. How often do recurrent attacks of herpes occur?

Nearly one-third of those who experienced an initial attack of herpes will never experience recurrent attacks. The virus can hibernate indefinitely. On the other hand, some individuals suffer from years of repeated episodes. Although subsequent attacks are usually briefer, milder and increasingly farther apart, occasionally certain victims have more frequent, severe attacks. It is not yet known why the course of herpes differs from individual to individual. Two forces seem to be at work: the strength of the body's immune defense system and the virulence of the particular strain of infecting virus. There is persuasive evidence some strains are particularly weak; others, exceptionally virulent.

42. Between attacks, can an infected person safely have sex?

Yes, but certain protective measures should be taken. These are discussed in detail in Part IV of this book.

43. May two people with genital herpes safely have sexual relations with each other when active lesions are present?

No, not unless both have the same type of virus, the same strain of the virus, in exactly the same areas of the body, and they make sure that no infected area touches an uninfected area of the other's body. Quite an improbable scenario. The potential for same-strain infection at different sites and the potential for different-strain infection at both the same and different sites is a much greater potential between two persons with herpes than is the fourth possibility, same-strain, same exact site. Indeed, this latter is somewhat akin to lightning striking twice in the same place; chances are it won't. Therefore, any feelings of security two people may have from the knowledge they both are herpes carriers are strictly false.

44. Can genital herpes be acquired by nonsexual means?

This is highly unlikely as the herpes virus is unable to survive for very long when away from the human body.

45. Can herpes be contracted from a toilet seat?

Theoretically yes; practically, possible but highly unlikely. Recent experiments have resulted in the successful culture of the herpes virus from an inanimate object after 72 hours following contact between the object and a volunteer subject's active herpes lesion. This is unlike both syphilis and gonorrhea, both of which die quickly in an atmosphere other than that of their natural host.* Much doubt exists within the scientific community whether anyone has ever contracted herpes from a toilet seat. In fact, with genital herpes, one would have to be somewhat of a gymnast to assume a posture which would permit contact between the usual sites of genital lesions and the toilet seat. Notwithstanding, it still is good hygienic practice to place toilet paper over the seat when using a public toilet.

Wet or moist fabrics, particularly towels and washclothes, are much more likely to transmit herpes. The virus thrives in warm moist areas. It can not survive on clean, dry fabrics.

> *Note:* Public panic was aroused with the announcement of this research, confusing theory with practical occurrence. Obvious precautions should be taken — not using towels or washclothes belonging to an individual with herpes and not sharing his or her toothbrush or eating utensils — but the implications of the one study should not be exaggerated.

46. Can herpes be caught in a swimming pool or hot tub?

No. Herpes is destroyed easily by heat exceeding normal

body temperature and is readily inactivated by chemicals used in pools. Herpes does not survive for long after leaving the body anyway.

47. Can herpes be caught from a pet?

Only if it is a person who is kept as a pet. Each animal species has its own virus or viruses to which it exclusively is susceptible. A cat's herpes or a dog's herpes cannot infect a human contact, and vice-versa. Humans are the only carriers of herpes simplex virus HSV-1 and HSV-2.

48. What is the most common clinical form of herpes?

Of all the forms of herpes recurrent herpes of the lips is the most common type seen clinically. The herpes blisters almost always appear and recur in the same location along the outer border of one of the lips. The onset of an attack is characterized by a burning or stinging sensation, and pain around the site of infection. With a severe attack the lymph nodes of the neck — the glands which drain the involved area — become swollen as the blisters form. Typically, the recurrences have been taking place for many years at the same site and the diagnosis does not present any problem. Rarely the lesions are confused with trench mouth or lip cancer.

If there is any doubt the diagnosis is made by the physician taking a scraping from the lesion and staining the scrapings. Interestingly, the staining test also would produce a positive result from the scrapings of chickenpox or shingles lesions. Of course, the clinical picture — the location on the lip of the blister and the accompanying symptomatology — avoids confusion. Generally the lesions are mild and self-limiting. Rarely, however, they can be severe and disfiguring.

49. How does herpes affect the eyes?

Herpes of the eyes most frequently affects the cornea — the clear portion overlying the lens of the eye (Fig. 6). The disease is called herpes keratitis. Conscientious care is highly important once an infection occurs, for herpetic keratitis is the most frequent cause of *infectious* blindness in the United States. This possible dire consequence occurs only when the condition is neglected, and the condition does not exist without definite symptoms. While it *can* affect both eyes, this occurs only when the virus is spread externally to the second eye.

Occasionally, herpes keratitis attacks as a primary infection. As noted earlier, herpes of the lips remains dormant in the trigeminal nerve ganglion. When reactivated, the virus can take, so to speak, a "wrong fork in the road". Rather than following the nerve from the trigeminal ganglion to the lip, it will follow a nerve path from the trigeminal ganglion to the eye. This is possible because the nerves serving the eyes are rooted in close proximity to the nerves serving the lips. As might be expected, herpes of the eye frequently is accompanied by herpes of the lips. Similarly, in most adults such infections are HSV-1. It is when the condition occurs in newborns that the infection is likely to be HSV-2, because the newborn will contract the disease as it passes through its mother's cervix and vagina during the process of birth.

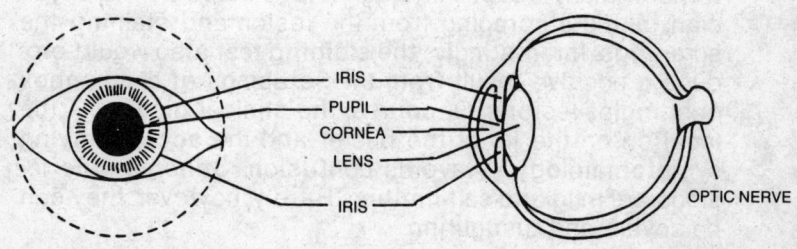

Fig. 6 – Eye

The most common source of herpes keratitis is self-inoculation. Believe it or not, many persons moisten their contact lenses with their saliva. This is a most unhygienic practice and should be avoided at all costs by a person who has herpes — even when the virus is not, or is not thought to be, active. Rubbing the eyes after the hands have been in contact with the virus is a source of infection, as is drying the face with a towel which has been in contact with an infected area of the body. A good rule to follow is to use separate towels when bathing; one for the body and one for the face. The body should be dried first. The hands should be washed thoroughly and then the face should be dried, drying the area around the eyes before any other part of the face is allowed to contact the towel.

Initially, herpes keratitis resembles ordinary "pink eye". The irritation in the eye increases. Persons with this condition often feel as though there is a foreign body in their eye, particularly in the upper lid. Painful sensitivity to light, called photophobia may develop. The eye may tear (*teer,* or weep) a watery material or may discharge mucus.

Following the initial stages of the attack, ulcers begin to form on the cornea. This is accompanied by an aching pain. After the cornea has become ulcerated, the next site of infection will be the iris. A continued absence of treatment may lead to glaucoma or to the formation of cataracts.

In the past, herpetic keratitis was treated by scraping the ulcers. Today, however, effective drugs are available for the treatment of the disease.

50. Does herpes sometimes infect the throat?

Yes. Almost exclusively from oral-genital sexual contact, herpes of the throat occurs as a complication of primary genital herpes. Symptoms of this complication include sore throat, fever, tonsillitis with exudate and swollen glands in the neck. Any woman who engages in oral-genital sexual activity and subsequently develops difficulty urinating together with a sore throat, should be aware of the likelihood of genital herpes lesions in her pelvis. (Genital lesions in males are usually external and obvious.)

51. What is herpes eczema?

Herpes eczema occurs when the herpes virus is superimposed upon an extensive pre-existing skin condition, one characterized by raw, open surfaces which naturally would be vulnerable to viral infestation. At times, the opportunity for rapid and extensive viral spreading may be offered by an allergic or atopic dermatitis. This form of herpes eczema can be life-threatening, and the use of intravenous acyclovir or experimental drugs may be mandatory if fatal consequences are to be averted.

It is interesting to note that while those with atopic dermatitis are more prone to herpes of the skin, those with psoriasis seem to be resistant to both herpes and superimposed bacterial infections at the site of their psoriatic lesions.

52. What is herpes meningitis?

Sometimes, when a recurrence of genital herpes begins, and the virus starts to travel from the sacral ganglia to the external genital area, the virus journeys "off course". It ends up on the meninges: the membranes which cover the brain and spinal cord. Since most genital infections are HSV-2, so are most cases of this type of herpes meningitis.

Herpes meningitis also can originate from the trigeminal ganglia, when a recurrence of "above the waist" herpes begins. The process is the same as that described above, except that it is the meninges which cover the brain that end up being infected by the virus. As expected, this kind of herpes meningitis most often is an HSV-1 infection; although, if the original oral infection were HSV-2, so would be the meningeal infection.

Herpes meningitis produces dramatic, and, at times, alarming, symptoms. Fever and varying degrees of mental confusion are among them. When the meningitis is trigeminal in origin, symptoms also include severe headache, stiffness in the neck, nausea and vomiting. In spite of the severe symptoms of the disorder, herpes meningitis is benign and self-limited. It does not cause other, serious neurological conditions; there are no convulsions and consciousness is not lost. Treatment for herpes meningitis is supportive only — rest, increasing fluid intake and analgesics. Complete recovery without complications or sequelae is the rule.

53. What is herpes encephalitis?

A herpes infection of the brain is called herpes encephalitis. Unlike herpes meningitis, herpes encephalitis is deadly. Fortunately, it is as rare as it is lethal, attacking an estimated one person in every million persons with herpes per year. The mortality rate from herpes of the brain is 50 to 70%. Often those who survive are left with serious, permanent residual defects (i.e. brain damage). What makes herpes encephalitis even more dangerous is the difficulty in making the diagnosis. The only group in whom the condition is diagnosed easily are newborn infants. In newborns, the combination of visible external lesions and the presence of central nervous system symptoms facilitates diagnosis.

Herpes encephalitis can come from both primary attacks and recurrent attacks of herpes. Herpes encephalitis is not associated with genital herpes! As the virus travels from the infection site to the trigeminal ganglion, it strays "off course", as it does with herpes meningitis. Instead of attacking the membranes covering the brain, though, the virus attacks the brain itself. Since herpes encephalitis occurs as the virus travels up the olfactory nerve to the brain instead of to the trigeminal ganglion, it usually is associated with oral, labial or facial herpes and similarly is usually an HSV-1 infection. Why or how the virus can take such an odd path, and end up in the brain, is unknown.

54. How is herpes encephalitis treated?

Adenenine arabinoside, also known both as Ara-A or vidarabine, is specific for treating herpes encephalitis. The drug is sold under the trade name of Vira-A. Ara-A is administered over a period of several hours through an intravenous drip. The drug is not given orally, intramuscularly or subcutaneously, for these routes of administration do not result in the body absorbing the drug well.

55. Is Ara-a useful for genital herpes?

No. The risk/benefit ratio of the current form of the drug is too high to permit its use except in life-threatening situations.

56. Are other forms of Ara-a helpful for herpes skin infections?

No. Various preparations containing Ara-A have been designed to be applied to the skin. In many clinical trials, these skin preparations have been shown *not* effective for treating genital or oral herpes. However, these same preparations have been proved useful for herpes *eye* infections. Research studies have shown Ara-A to be effective in the treatment of congenital herpes, but this use is still experimental.

Skin preparations containing Ara-C or Ara-AMP, which are both close relatives of Aar-A, have also been proved *not* effective against herpes skin infections.

57. Does herpes sometimes involve the digestive tract?

In rare instances, herpes can infect the esophagus, the tube leading from the mouth to the stomach. Because it is rare, herpes of the esophagus may be confused with a bleeding peptic ulcer or with varicosities of the esophageal veins, such as those seen in cases of cirrhosis. Esophageal herpes should always be considered in the differential diagnosis of diseases that cause upper gastro-intestinal symptoms.

Some of the more common diseases which could account for some or most of the symptoms of herpes of the esophagus are various ulcers, hiatus hernia, gall bladder disease and coronary insufficiency.

During the acute phase of esophageal herpes, both in the initial attack and in recurrences, heartburn and difficulty in swallowing may be present. Occasionally, there may be episodes of bleeding. While that sounds dramatic, esophageal herpes is, like other forms of herpes, self-limiting, and usually resolves without any untoward problems.

58. Is there such a thing as chronic herpes simplex skin lesions?

Yes. The condition is called chronic (over a long period of time) cutaneous herpes simplex. While most cases of herpes resolve themselves within two weeks, an episode of persistant herpetic ulcer may go on for months at a time.

Chronic cutaneous herpes simplex generally occurs only in those individuals whose immunological systems are deficient. The body's immunological system can be affected adversely by debilitation or a chronically debilitating illness. The use of anti-cancer medication or other immuno-suppressive drugs, such as those used in organ transplant cases to prevent rejection of the donor organ, also can make the body vulnerable to persistent herpetic ulcer.

Though rare, some cases of chronic recurrent herpes have been reported in otherwise healthy persons. Presumably, in such a case the individual has an immunological problem. Any person whose immunological defenses are compromised is prey not only to herpes but to any number of opportunistic, parasitic organisms.

The greatest danger of persistent herpetic ulcer is the presence of chronically active, destructive skin lesions, which have the potential to spread and become disseminated systematically into the body.

Intravenous Acyclovir has been approved for use in the chronic ulcerating disease in those whose immunological systems are poor. The results of this form of therapy have been quite encouraging.

59. Does herpes sometimes infect the fingers?

Herpes simplex infections of the finger are called whitlows. They are caused by HSV-2 slightly more often than they are by HSV-1. When the tips of the fingers become infected, the ulcers around the fingernails are red and swollen. Often herepetic whitlow is not diagnosed, and treatment is initiated for what appears to be a bacterial paronychia. Antibiotics are prescribed — which, as with all forms of herpes viruses, don't help — and the incisions made to drain the sores (i.e. of what mistakenly is thought to be a paronychia) only make the condition worse, by prolonging the healing time of the lesions. Accurate diagnosis, then, is important. More than half the cases of herpetic whitlow may be regarded as incidents of sexually transmitted disease.

60. Are medical personnel at risk for catching herpes infections?

Almost ironically, it is health care professionals who are most vulnerable to herpetic whitlow. Dentists, for instance, routinely are exposed to the virus, as are their hygienists. Doctors, nurses and respiratory therapists, can contract the disease during examinations and other procedures in which there is contact with the patients. Usually this occurs when herpes is not suspected, and thus no precautionary measure, such as wearing rubber gloves, is taken. When the sores of oral herpes are present, a person may also shed virus in his saliva. Dental personnel should be aware of this phenomenon and take precautions.

61. Who usually contracts acute herpes of the mouth and gums?

This form of herpes is seen most often in children five years of age and younger. Up through that age, the immunological defense system is not developed sufficiently to bring the infection under control without a prolonged and severe battle. Any portion of the oral cavity can be involved. Such an attack is characterized by red swollen gums with blisters on the mucous membranes of the mouth accompanied by high fever, pain and fetid breath. The lymph nodes under the chin — the submaxillary glands — become swollen. Occasionally, the infection may become so pronounced the child is unable to eat or to drink. Dehydration then becomes a real danger; and without proper treatment the condition can be a potential threat to life. In rare instances, the disease may involve the larynx (vocal chords), causing an obstruction in the airway and necessitating immediate emergency medical care. Acute herpes of the mouth and gums is seen in adults, following oral-genital sexual activity when the partner has genital lesions.

PART III:
Diagnosing Herpes

62. Should a person consult a physician if he or she suspects genital herpes?

Yes, it is important to see a physician as soon as possible. Only a physician can determine whether or not you have genital herpes. Diagnosis of the herpes type, however, can only be made when the sores are present.

63. How are herpes simplex virus infections usually diagnosed?

Herpes infections may be diagnosed by a physician who recognizes the characteristic sores. Sometimes it is difficult to diagnose herpes on the basis of appearance alone. Many patients report to their physician after the vesicles have ruptured and only ulcerations are visible, thus partially obscuring the chance for the physician to observe the lesions in their classical form. The clinical diagnosis of herpes — diagnosis from appearance only — is the least reliable method for diagnosing the disease. Without laboratory tests, *absolute* certainty in diagnosis can not be attained and more harm than good results when herpes is misdiagnosed. Laboratory tests are extremely useful whenever there is doubt or when unquestionable accuracy is demanded by the circumstances. Certainly in the case of a pregnant female it is imperative the diagnosis be wholly reliable; for, should the tests prove positive, it is crucial to monitor the activity of the infection throughout the entire term of pregnancy.

Most major cities have virology laboratories, where the culturing of viruses is conducted. In rural or suburban areas, the cell swabs or scrapings can be kept on ice for two to three days. This is ample time for the specimen to be shipped to a virology laboratory and cultured there.

The process of growing the virus in the artificial environment of the laboratory is called culturing. Tissue cells known to be good host cells are grown in the laboratory. These cells are inoculated with specimens obtained from the suspected areas of viral infestation. (If the virus does indeed grow on the tissue, the culture is said to be positive. Should the virus not grow on the tissue, it presumably means the tissue contained no virus in the first place. The culture is then said to be negative.) Although the virus itself is never visible in a tissue culture, the destructive effects of the virus on the host cells is clearly apparent. When these destructive effects occur, the culture is said to be positive. When they do not occur, and no alteration in the host cells is noted, the culture is said to be negative. It should be noted that even in the presence of obvious lesions and the employment of proper techniques for culturing, cultures will not be 100% reliable. In one large university study of prenatal monitoring, cultures were positive in only 40% of the cases, despite obvious clinical evidence to the contrary.

Cytology is the science dealing with the nature of cells. The destructive effects upon the host cells of the virus in a positive culture are called cytopathic effects. With such cytopathic effects, in conjunction with knowledge of the source of the specimen with which the laboratory host cells were inoculated, with knowledge of the type of host cellular tissue used in the culture and with an evaluation of the rate at which the cytopathic effects occur, a reliable diagnosis can be made.

64. Can a blood test be used to diagnose herpes?

Yes, but it is an indirect method of diagnosis.

65. What does a positive blood test mean?

If a blood sample is analyzed, the lab will test for the presence of *antibodies* to herpes simplex virus and not for the virus itself. If specific antibodies are found, it is assumed that (1) the patient has, at some time, been exposed, to herpes simplex virus, and (2) because of this exposure, his or her body has made antibodies against the virus. Such antibodies may remain in the blood for years after the original infection, even if it produced no symptoms in the patient. A positive blood test means that a person has *or* has had a herpes simplex virus infection at some time in the past. In other words, someone who once had herpes but who has not experienced a recurrence for many years and who now is not experiencing a recurrence may still have a higher antibody titer in his bloodstream than a person who never has had herpes at all. For this reason, repeated serum viral titer tests must be done. Only if the titer rises appreciably after an interval of time can it be said a new infection of the disease is present.

66. Can a blood test be used to type the herpes simplex virus?

Yes, but it is an indirect method that is not always accurate. Blood antibodies can be typed. However, in some tests, antibodies to Type 2 behave as if they were antibodies to Type 1 and vice versa. Therefore, unless very sensitive procedures are used, it may be impossible to tell, on the basis of blood antibodies alone, exactly which strain of herpes simplex virus a person has or has had.

67. How can the exact type of herpes simples virus (Type 1 or Type 2) be determined?

The two types produce identical clinical sores and identical patterns in the Tzanck smear. However, they have different patterns of viral growth, and may be distinguished in a viral culture.

In a research lab, special reagents may be available to type the virus by immunochemical methods. These techniques differentiate Type 1 from Type 2 on the basis of different proteins located on the outside of each virus.

The most reliable way to differentiate Types 1 and 2 is to analyze the DNA (deoxyribonucleic acid) or genetic material of the virus.

68. Is the typing of herpes easy to do?

No. Unfortunately, the average clinical lab is not prepared to do this test and the special equipment needed for herpes typing usually are stocked only by research or reference laboratories.

69. Is it important to know what type of herpes virus is involved in a case of genital herpes?

Not really. While typing can be conducted in the laboratory, there is not much, if any, practical benefit to be derived as a result of differentiating between the two basic types of herpes infections. Whether HSV-1 or HSV-2, both treatment and outlook will be the same. Some experimental drugs appear to be type specific but this is, as yet, of no practical importance.

Studies have shown, though, that HSV-1 of the genital area is less likely to recur than is HSV-2. Notwithstanding these studies it must be remembered that both Type 1 and Type 2 can be transmitted both orally and genitally; and that when laboratory typing is done, it is done after and not before the fact.

70. Can a pap smear help diagnose genital herpes?

The *pap smear* is named after the medical scientist who developed it — Dr. George Papanicolaou. Usually associated with the detection of cervical cancer in women, the pap smear also is effective in detecting herpes, both of the cervix and of other sites on the body. The pap smear will not differentiate between the two herpes simplex viruses.

A pap smear accurately diagnoses genital herpes in about two-thirds of the cases. In the other third, it results in a false negative diagnosis.

Smear tests are interpreted by a pathologist, a physician whose specialty is the study of the nature of diseases by means of tissue examination. In the case of herpes, the pathologist's study is conducted microscopically. Smear tests are indirect tests. Under the microscope, the virus itself is not seen, but rather the characteristic appearance caused by the virus is noted. A positive test reveals multi-nucleated giant cells with distinctive intra-nuclear inclusions within the host cells.

The cytologist reading the pap smear should be alerted to the possibility of a herpes infection, and a search made for the characteristic cells associated with the disease. In other words, the identification should not be relied upon as an incidental finding during a routine pap smear.

PART IV:
Prevention and Control of Herpes

71. Is there any surefire way to prevent herpes?

Yes. Avoid all physical contact with other persons. Short of such drastic action, nothing is "sure" but the 1-2-3 program is a more practical approach.

1. **Active Disease:** Abstain completely.
2. **Between Recurrences:** Condom, contraceptive foam or gel plus diaphragm.
3. **Decrease Promiscuity:** Preferably one partner only.

Any individual who suspects that he or she has herpes should use, or have the partner use a condom, and/or diaphragm when having sexual relations. The regular use of condoms by males and diaphragms by females is a safe procedure to adopt, especially when used with contraceptive foam or spermicidal jelly. The foam and jellies which were designed to kill sperm, also can kill the herpes virus. However, contraceptive jellies cannot be relied upon completely for protection as there is still some controversy as to the level of effectiveness in killing the herpes virus. Condoms do not cover the scrotum, thighs, buttocks or abdomen, common sites of infection, and diaphragms also can not be relied upon to seal off and protect the cervix.

72. If one is unwilling to follow the strict 1-2-3 program outlined previously, what constitutes a reasonable compromise program to protect the uninfected partner?

Contracting the virus from one's partner is, for practical purposes, tantamount to contact with the partner's active lesions. To the extent this can be avoided, the chances of protecting the uninfected partner are good. Both persons, especially the infected one, must become very astute at recognizing the reactivation of the virus from its earliest signs. It is important to notice the onset of the prodrome since the virus can be shed during this period, even prior to the eruption of lesions. Of course, total abstinence must be practiced from the time the very first prodromal symptom is noticed until the recurrence has abated entirely.

Since the virus can not be spread in its dormant phase, this question really comes down to how does one know when the virus is active?

The only sure tangible sign of activity is the presence of lesions. Because as noted, some persons shed the virus without the presence of physical symptoms, and, since the idea of having cultures done one or more times daily — the most reliable means of ascertaining the virus' activity — is absurd, a compromise protection program for one's partner is best accomplished upon a basis of circumstances being either "more likely" or "less likely" to result in infection. And, sure as the sun rises in the east and sets in the west, circumstances will be evaluated by whether or not the physical symptoms are there.

Between the absolute presence and the absolute absence of physical symptoms — lesions — is a certain amount of grey area. Has one recently had experiences which, when similar experiences were had in past, were or customarily are followed by recurrences? Thus, each individual's somewhat unique viral history becomes important, which is why a person can not be too aware of the particular way the virus behaves in him or her.

At such times, when "less likely" and "more likely" are not easily distinguished from each other, a better-safe-than-sorry approach should be taken. In practical terms, this means minimizing intimate contact and taking the few available precautions when intimate contact occurs. Regardless of who the carrier is, both partners should institute the 1-2-3 barrier program previously outlined. Avoid oral-genital contact and hand-to-genital contact until "less likely" clearly emerges again.

73. If one partner has genital herpes, what are the other partner's chances of contracting the disease, given repeated exposure?

In spite of the fact precautions may be taken, and in spite

of the fact many couples are conscientious in taking them, the chances of the uninfected partner eventually contracting genital herpes remain relatively high. A study of a large group of persons whose spouses had genital herpes revealed 50 to 60% of the uninfected partners contracted the disease. The study did not last forever; therefore, with time, that percentage figure can only go up, not down.

Be that as it may, many partners of persons with herpes never develop the disease. This probably is a result of both good hygienic practices and good individual resistance to the virus.

Remaining free of the disease over the years when the partner has genital herpes and when sexual activity is routine certainly is possible and many persons are proof of this possibility.

Generally, the possibility of contracting genital herpes is not sufficient grounds to terminate an otherwise rewarding relationship.

74. What are the advantages of having only one sexual partner?

If neither party has herpes, fidelity between them is the best safeguard against the disease. Even if one or both partners have herpes, dealing effectively with the disease is measurably facilitated if the relationship is enduring and closed.

In the case in which one or both have herpes and the relationship is long-term and the partners are faithful to each other, many advantages are gained. A regimen of barrier protection is initiated and maintained more easily. The partners are more familiar, and continue to become increasingly familiar, with each other's bodies. Thus, recurrences are noticed at their earliest stages. However, the most important factor is the intimate interpersonal relationship the two share. The openness, understanding and communication such a relationship permits is the couple's most potent tool for coping with the condition, especially with the mental aspects of the condition.

As the number of sexual partners a person has increases

and as the length of relationships decreases, the above advantages dwindle proportionately.

75. Will washing and urinating immediately following sexual relations also help to prevent herpes?

Washing with hot, soapy water right after sexual activity will reduce the chance of getting any sexually transmitted disease, including herpes. *However,* washing removes only those virus particles that have not yet penetrated the cells or gained entry otherwise, such as through the urethral channel; *and,* there is no guarantee washing will remove *all* virus particles still on the surface of the skin. Viruses invade rapidly, and no amount of scrubbing will prevent infection once cellular penetration by the virus has occurred.

This does not discount the simple fact washing is a good hygienic practice. So, while not to be overestimated, neither should washing be underestimated. Though it offers no protection against cervical or vaginal infection, washing indeed may prevent vulvar and penile infection. Wherever the virus lies superficially, washing has the *potential* to cleanse the body of the virus in those areas.

The problem is many especially vulnerable areas of the body are not easily accessible to washing, and much infection occurs *during* sexual relations. What occurs *during* sexual activity usually can not be reversed *following* sexual activity — immediately or otherwise.

Notwithstanding, urinating following intercourse can wash out any viral particles which may have entered the urethra but not yet penetrated the cells lining the urethral channel. This procedure is recommended equally for males and females as one of several precautionary steps. The preventive steps must be taken together in order to significantly reduce the chances of contracting the virus. Of course, the only sure preventive measure which is effective alone is abstinence — not a very pleasant way to avoid an unpleasant problem.

76. What can be done to reduce the incidence or recurrent attacks?

Tight clothing, including tight undergarments or pantyhose, can be a contributing factor in the reactivation of the virus. Synthetic undergarments are to be avoided. When the first prodromal symptom of a recurrence is noticed, men may wish to wear cotton boxer-style shorts and women may wish not to wear panties. Women who develop a vaginal discharge may wear a minipad. When retiring for the night, it is advisable to sleep in the nude. For those whose custom it is to sleep in the nude anyway, the mate may wish to wear pajamas or some form of nightshirt or gown, to eliminate the risk of rubbing against a contagious lesion.

In all cases it is of paramount importance to avoid scratching, despite the severity of the itching or burning. If one catches oneself having scratched automatically, the hands should be washed as soon as possible, and certainly before any other area of the body is touched.

Again, at the first prodromal symptom, even when it is only a slight tingling, all sexual contact should cease completely until every lesion which may subsequently develop has been gone for at least the better part of a week. Steady partners should be frank and open with each other, and not hesitate to examine one another for early evidence of lesions. Often another can spot what may be physically difficult for oneself to notice.

Know at least the more common factors which can incite a recurrent attack. These include physical stress, mental stress or distress, menstruation, smoking, exposure to ultraviolet light rays (such as sunlight), sexual activity, infections in the body and other conditions that can lower the body's general resistance.

Emotional stress and anxiety can be relieved by the prescription of a tranquilizer by a qualified physician; although the preferred method of dealing with stress is to adjust one's social and vocational life so that undue stress, especially when it becomes distress, is avoided. Admittedly, this can not always be done easily, and unfortunately for many, such adjustments just are too impractical to attempt — and attempting them may lead only to further stress as the attempt fails. Moderate exercise, such as jogging, and light, disciplined exercises, such as those yoga comprises, can help to eliminate, control or reduce physical stress.

Premenstrual tension often can be relieved by the appropriate prescription of a diuretic. Effective sunscreens are abundantly available on the market, and prolonged or over-exposure to the sun's rays is avoided simply enough by wearing a broad-brimmed hat or by going indoors. Remember: the brightness of the sun or the heat of the day are not reliable measures of ultraviolet rays. Ultraviolet rays can penetrate what are called "overcast skies" and can even be reflected by snow.

When suffering from infection or when otherwise "under the weather", the steps recommended by one's physician that will lead to the speediest possible recovery should be followed to the letter.

Lastly, a realistic attitude toward herpes in general and recurrences in particular should be adopted. Constant dread and fear of a recurrence can become a self-fulfilling prophecy and lead to a vicious cycle: causing a recurrence, which in turn intensifies one's anxieties, which in turn causes more frequent or more severe recurrences, or both.

Good personal hygiene is very important, yet anything can be carried to excess. Some persons with herpes become nothing short of compulsive. They emulate Lady Macbeth, repeatedly washing their hands to the point their hands become chapped. They change towels and sheets with much greater frequency than necessary. The precautions one takes to prevent herpes recurrences must not be permitted to develop into fetishes. Just as important as taking intelligent measures to avoid outbreaks of the virus is avoiding turning those measures into rituals. Herpes must be seen in perspective, in toto.

The person with herpes can learn to live with it. And, since he has no other choice but *to* live with it, he is fortunate at least in that respect, and a proper perspective on his condition will go a long way toward minimizing the problems of his condition.

77. Do people sometimes become confused about who caught what from whom?

Sexual activity is thought to be the most common trigger of recurrent herpes episodes. That is, the physical act of sex triggers the reactivation of the dormant virus, not that sexual activity triggers new viral infection. This can be a most distressing problem and occasionally leads to much unfortunate confusion, for an individual may mistake a recurrence with a reinfection, and the finger of accusation may be pointed without just cause.

This is commonly seen when a person who has been abstinent for a long period of time meets a new sexual companion, then experiences a recurrent attack of herpes; then, the herpes being reactivated infects the companion. Both parties feel adamantly each has contracted herpes from the other, with the companion, the "innocent" party, bearing the brunt of the misunderstanding. Since both will culture positively, testing proves nothing, yet is likely to entrench the first person in his or her misperception of the companion further.

To compound the problem at least two percent of women and one percent of men with herpes shed the virus between attacks, without any tangible signs. The greatest problems, though, are likely to be experienced by the person whose initial attack of herpes (which may have occurred years earlier) was asymptomatic: nothing can convince him his first recurrence is not an initial infection. Thus the sudden appearance of herpes in a marriage or long term relationship does not invariably imply infidelity. As if all this were not enough, it must be remembered that oral sex is a form of sexual activity and so has the same potential for triggering recurrences or causing genital herpes as does intercourse.

At times, circumstances can combine (as if in a conspiracy) in such a manner that the underlying facts never can be reliably ascertained. It is important to demonstrate understanding rather than hostility to those less aware and who do jump to such conclusions. Once again, the interpersonal consequences of herpes can be far more devastating than the physical consequences of the disease.

78. What is the role of sex education in schools in herpes prevention?

There still are many persons in this country who oppose so-called "sex education classes" in school. These people believe such classes promote, or at least grant tacit approval to, sexual activity between adolescent partners or, in some cases, promiscuity among adolescents. The sex education debate is hardly a new one. Its introduction into most high school curricula has been and has remained controversial from the start. It is most unfortunate that the opposition to sex education classes has stemmed from moral judgments about the tendencies these classes instill in students. Whatever adolescents do or don't do about sexual activity — which, after a number of years of sex education being taught, seems to bear little or no relationship to the existence of such classes — the dangers of sexually transmitted disease are very real in the world in which students and adults both live.

These dangers are met only by awareness and knowledge of them, which is best gained by education. In the case of sexually transmitted diseases, experience often is a cruel teacher, and even more often a poor teacher. By all indications, the greatest protection from sexually transmitted diseases is a joint effort between school and parent: real and useful information from the former and realistic and compassionate guidance from the latter.

Sexual activity among adolescents has never been and never will be confined to delinquents. Intelligent, sincere, honest young men and women — who happen to be or, at worst, simply believe themselves to be, in love — become parents and contract sexually transmitted diseases. It takes no more than a single sexual encounter for either to occur. To whatever moral discipline one adheres — in whatever way the "downside" of affirmative, sex education programs is perceived — the consequence of sexual activity among adolescents in an uninformed ignorant atmosphere are far worse.

Any given sexually active single person, it being immaterial whether he or she is over or under 18 years of age, has a better than fair chance of contracting a sexually transmitted disease within a year's time. Education, and the openness between partners it inspires, is the best insurance of early diagnosis and the early institution of treatment, and in all probability the best future defense against such a sorry statistic.

PART V:
Treatments for Herpes

79. What ineffective "cures" for herpes have been touted?

Herpes is a disease the course of which often proves erratic. The exacerbations and remissions of herpes can be highly unpredictable. In terms of severity, duration and frequency of recurrence, the disease can vary significantly from individual to individual.

Many different so-called "cures" for herpes have been touted. It has been "suggested" by some that there exists a gigantic conspiracy on the part of the medical community to conceal and withhold from the public acknowledgement of the particular cure for herpes which a particular advocate proclaims. Contrary to what many food faddists and impressionable persons may believe, such a conspiracy is pure fiction. The medical community is one of the most open communities in the world. Without regard to politics, economics or nationality, physicians and medical researchers everywhere freely exchange knowledge and information daily, on a scale so wide and so vast it defies comprehension how such goodwill and cooperation can exist and be maintained in a world as plagued by troubles as is the one in which we live.

At one time or another, everything from Vitamin E to old fashioned snake venom has been advocated as a cure. Following anecdotal reports, Betadine soap, an excellent antiseptic, was used widely. Betadine soap does not cure herpes.

Dimethysulfoxide, commonly known as DMSO, a solvent reportedly helpful in treating certain rheumatic disorders, has been tried. Because of DMSO's ability to penetrate the intact skin and carry other substances with it in the process, it recently has been used as the transport vehicle for other medications. DMSO alone has no effect on herpes viruses.

In early 1979, dye light therapy was tried. This "treatment" consists of painting the involved area with a light-sensitive dye. The area is then exposed to ultraviolet light. Dye light therapy does not cure herpes. It also subsequently was discovered, in laboratory studies, dye light therapy could cause cancer.

For a while, the lay press touted lithium as a cure. Lithium does not cure herpes. Nevertheless, some herpes sufferers do claim that lithium decreases the severity and duration of their attacks. Lysine, a naturally occurring amino acid, present in large quantities in such foods as eggs, potatoes and milk, was shown in certain studies to prevent the virus from growing, under laboratory conditions. These same studies noted arginine, another amino acid, was required for the growth of the virus. Many persons claimed their lesions disappeared overnight and these persons did appear to do well on maintenance therapy. The author has had a number of patients who swore by lysine. Fine enough: dairy products, apart from their high cholesterol content, are healthy foods, and potatoes are an excellent complex carbohydrate source. However, after a period of time, the lysine seemed no longer to be be effective. While the first rule and requirement for any form of medical treatment was met — namely, above all do no harm — lysine fell somewhat short of meeting the second requirement: it did not affect herpes in controlled studies.

The list of attempted therapies goes on and on, and even includes the vaccines used for yellow fever and BCG.*
Curiously, though, a certain number of persons will, at least temporarily, appear to respond to treatments, scientifically known to be ineffective. No treatment consistently helps a broad variety of herpes victims, yet each treatment works for a while with some. What can explain this seemingly impossible paradox? The answer is the placebo effect.

> *Bacillus Calmette-Guerin vaccine which stimulates the production of antibodies against tuberculosis but is ineffective against herpes.

80. What is the placebo effect?

The human mind is a tremendous storehouse of power, most of it unrealized and unappreciated. Some of the mind's fantastic abilities are easily demonstrated when summoned under hypnosis. For instance an hypnotized individual can keep his arm raised above his head for hours without feeling the least bit tired or strained. He will experience no muscle fatigue or alterations in his metabolism. Waking, alert persons would experience great fatigue and metabolic changes and would be unable to duplicate the feat.

The author recalls performing a surgical operation on a subject, using hypnosis but no chemical anesthesia whatever. Upon suggesting to the patient that his bleeding stop, his autonomic nervous system responded by constricting his blood vessels leaving the operative field dry. He felt no pain from the scalpel or from the stitching. The effects of hypnosis have been widely known for well over a century. While suggestion always is involved, to call hypnosis mere suggestion is a gross understatement and says nothing.

It is thought by most scientists that whatever makes hypnosis work also accounts for what is called the placebo effect. The same sort of phenomena which occur when a hypnotist makes suggestions to a hypnotized subject can be seen in the waking state to a limited, lesser degree. Such waking suggestions can be self-induced, for the unconscious part of the human mind never is awake in the usual sense of the word.

Faith in a remedy is a form of waking hypnotic suggestion. It does not matter from where this faith comes. It may be a faith the individual has in another person who told him the remedy would work, it may be a faith the individual has in something he read, or it may be a wholly self-induced faith, based upon a strong wish. This is the major part of the placebo effect, and explains why the famous "sugar pill" often is effective against physical illness.

The placebo effect is not imaginary, as many persons believe. The patient taking lysine didn't "imagine" his lesions away any more than the hypnotized subject "imagines" he can hold his arm outstretched for hours. Both events occur in physical reality. They *happen.* The placebo effect accounts for different patients swearing by their different therapies, and why these therapies do not work in general for others. While a form of self-deception, what difference does it make if the belief of an individual serves to mobilize his defense system against viral infection?

Just as significantly, the unconscious portion of the mind can direct the body's functions to abort impending recurrences of herpes outbreaks.

81. What is Acyclovir?

A new antiviral drug called Acyclovir (trade name Zovirax) has been approved by the FDA for use against herpes simplex Types 1 and 2. In clinical trials of primary herpes genitalis, use of Acyclovir ointment resulted in a decrease in healing time and, in some cases, a decrease in pain and duration of viral shedding. In studies of recurrent genital herpes and oral herpes, there was no evidence of clinical benefit, although there was some decrease in duration of viral shedding.

Although Acyclovir affords some relief from primary herpes attacks, this topical medication is expensive: a small tube may cost $25.00. It also is messy and inconvenient, requiring up to six applications a day. For maximum effect the drug must be applied early in the course of the disease, preferably at the first sign of symptoms, even prior to the eruption of lesions. The home remedies are far less expensive and often are comparable to Acyclovir in symptom relief.

Acyclovir works not only on the skin, but can be administered intravenously in cases of life-threatening herpes infections. Though rare, such cases occur in chronically debilitated patients. This is the most important contribution of this medication to the physician's treatment arsenal. More convenient oral forms of Zovirax are currently being tested. The results of preliminary studies were reported in *The New England Journal of Medicine.* These reports are suggestive that capsules of Zovirax taken at the first sign of prodromal symptoms — tingling, burning, etc. — could possibly eliminate the recurrent outbreak. It has also been suggested that Zovirax might be of benefit orally to prevent recurrent attacks. The Burroughs Welcome Company, manufacturers of Zovirax, are awaiting approval from the FDA for the oral use of the medication.

A word of warning must be given to the promiscuous use of Acyclovir. The overuse, misuse or abuse of a drug like Acyclovir can lead to the development or evolution of resistant, mutant strains of the herpes virus. This is a genuine long-term risk with a potential that probably outweighs the minor, limited, immediate relief Acyclovir provides when used topically.

82. What other antiviral drugs are available?

Among the other drugs available to combat herpes is Bromovinyldeoxyuridine, or for short, BVDU. Like Acyclovir and Vidarabine, BVDU affects only those cells infected by the virus, leaving normal cells alone. The drug is effective particularly against HSV-1 and the chickenpox-booster virus. Its effectiveness against HSV-2 is minimal. The FDA has not approved BVDU for use in treating genital herpes, even though one-third of all cases of genital herpes in the 24 and under age bracket is HSV-1. FIAC is the abbreviation of another new drug, administered intravenously, that shows promise against both HSV-1 and HSV-2; and a number of other drugs is being investigated by researchers.

83. What is Interferon?

The antiviral agents discussed previously fall into the category of what are called *antimetabolites.* The most publicity, however, has surrounded another type of antiviral agent: *Interferon.*

Interferon is a natural antiviral agent. The body's white cells and fibroblasts manufacture Interferon in response to viral attacks. Infected host cells begin to excrete Interferon, which acts as a chemical messenger. Interferon informs uninfected, yet potential host cells of the invader; in this case, the herpes virus. The Interferon diffuses into nearby cells, or is transported by the body fluids. Upon receipt of the Interferon the uninfected cells protect themselves from viral attack. They accomplish this not by inhibiting penetration of the virus, but rather by preventing viral replication once penetration has occurred. (Thus, by itself, Interferon is not directly anti-viral.) The Interferon-treated potential host cells react chemically with the Interferon. The product of this chemical reaction is a second, new protein, called — appropriately — *anti-viral protein*. It is this, the anti-viral protein, which blocks viral replication when the Interferon-treated cell is invaded by the virus.

Until recently, Interferon was enormously expensive. With the rapid growth in the field of genetic engineering, researchers have been able to alter the DNA structure of certain common bacteria, according to a pre-determined plan, and turn the altered bacteria into a mass-production inexpensive source of Interferon.

A patient suffering from one viral infection usually does not contract another viral infection simultaneously. One virus seems to prevent another virus from successfully invading the body at the same time. The cells originally infected produce Interferon, a protein substance which notifies surrounding cells of the viral invader. Thus, when a neighboring cell is invaded, the Interferon released earlier advises the invaded cell to protect itself from the virus. Interferon displays a high theoretical potential for use against herpes infections. However, there are certain problems with its practical application. Several years ago, Interferon was heralded as a "wonder drug". It later was found that large doses of Interferon had some untoward effects. Contrary to initial speculation, Interferon now seems more effective when working in conjunction with the body's immune system, rather than being used as the sole factor for defense or for cure. While Interferon may yet prove a wonder drug, some disillusionment has followed the original sounding of the trumpets. All in all, though, Interferon is an amazing substance which may hold the keys to many doors in great need of opening.

84. What is the carbon dioxide laser treatment?

Another new treatment for herpes is the *carbon dioxide laser*. While this form of treatment is very expensive and not widely available, the carbon dioxide laser can give virtually instant relief to painful herpes lesions. It does this by vaporizing the lesions, without damaging any of the normal cells surrounding the lesions. It is said these laser treatments also increase the time between recurrences. Some researchers think if it were diagnosed and treatment with the laser begun in time, an outbreak of primary herpes could be arrested permanently and all recurrences prevented — that is, the condition could be cured. This, though possibly true, has not yet been proven in controlled studies over a period of time.

85. **Can herpes symptoms be relieved with simple home remedies?**

    Only to a limited extent. Generally the lesions should be kept dry, but bathing with soap and water is encouraged. Cold or ice compresses can have a soothing effect. Heat generally increases the pain of an attack. However, some female patients have reported relief and early cessation of recurrences with dry heat in the form of radiations from a light bulb in close proximity to the affected area. A goose neck lamp serves well for this purpose. This sort of heat application has been used for many years to help relieve the pain associated with the episiotomy sutures of childbirth. Compresses of a saline solution — a teaspoon of salt dissolved in a quart of water — can be used, and it is important to dry the infected area thoroughly afterward. Aspirin may help to relieve pain and fever. There are a number of over-the-counter medications available for herpes sufferers. Never use drugs containing steroids (e.g. cortisone) on a herpes lesion as it will worsen the problem and spread the virus.

    Special diets and nutritional supplements (e.g. zinc, lysine, vitamins, etc.) are not effective, many anecdotal stories to the contrary notwithstanding. Beware of the various claims made by sales persons intent on making money by false promotion of useless "herpes cures".

    For many years, physicians have recommended an *aqueous,* two percent solution of gentian violet for the treatment of aphthous ulcers in the mouth. The topical application of this solution is worth trying on herpes lesions — genital or oral.

    Be sure not to confuse the aqueous (in water) solution of gentian violet with the more common tincture, or alcohol, solution sold in most pharmacies.

    The topical application of milk of magnesia has been employed successfully as a pain reliever, too. (Yes, milk of magnesia is used more commonly as a laxative.) Allow the bottle to stand for several hours. The contents of the bottle will divide themselves into two sections. The clear supernatant (liquid portion) of the upper section should be poured away. It is the denser substances, which will have settled as the lower section, of the milk of magnesia that are applied, with a cotton swab, to the lesions. The effect is a desirable soothing and drying one.

86. Is the development of a vaccine against herpes close at hand?

It should not come as a surprise that the major pharmaceutical houses are devoting considerable time, effort and resources to cure or prevent a disease affecting 20 million persons. The health field is big business and an untold fortune awaits the corporation which secures the first patent on a safe and effective vaccine against the disease. Indeed, experimental vaccines have already been produced and are undergoing testing at the present time. Research proceeds daily, and will continue to do so until its goals — prevention and cure — are achieved.

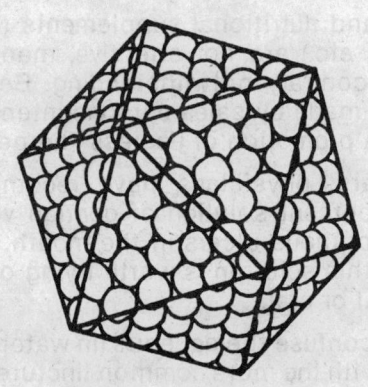

PART VI:
Herpes and Pregnancy

87. May a pregnant woman engage in intercourse, without special considerations, if either she or her partner has or develops herpes?

At any time during the term of pregnancy when the virus is active, sexual activity should be avoided. Premature deliveries are slightly more common in women with active herpes than in other women. Most physicians advise against sexual activity after the first seven months. The reason for this is an indirect one: sexual activity is a very common trigger for causing recurrent outbreaks of the virus. Thus, this is a preventive measure to insure no reactivation occurs in the latter stages of pregnancy or at the time of delivery.

Essentially the same precautions are to be taken when the woman's partner has herpes. When his infection is active, intimate contact must be avoided: *all* intimate contact, not just intercourse. When the male's infection is active, oral-genital and hand-to-genital contact likewise are to be avoided. The problems posed by the male's herpes exist only to the extent his infection can be transmitted to the woman.

And, as always, women should never douche when they are pregnant.

88. What kind of herpes infection in a pregnant woman is potentially dangerous to the unborn child?

Genital herpes, especially a first infection when there is greater opportunity for the virus to linger in the mother's genital area or to form a large pool for potential spread. It is not certain what effect herpes may have early in pregnancy. There may be no adverse effect if the virus is no longer present when the baby is being born. Only one study has found some association between a first infection of genital herpes during the first three months of pregnancy and a slightly increased rate of spontaneous abortion.

89. What may happen if a woman gets genital herpes for the first time late in pregnancy?

If the mother's first herpes infection occurs during the last three months of pregnancy, there is a possibility that the virus will remain in the genital tract up until the time of birth. If so, the child would be born through an infected birth canal and might become infected during birth. If herpes simplex is present in the genital tract of a pregnant woman near the time of delivery, her physician usually will plan a caesarean section (Fig. 7).

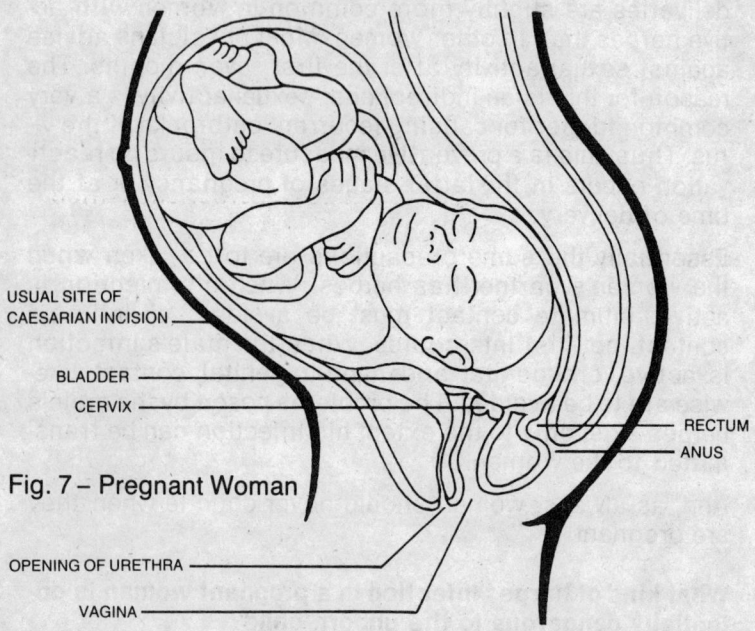

Fig. 7 – Pregnant Woman

90. How great a special danger does herpes pose to the newborn?

Thousands of women with *dormant* genital herpes give birth vaginally to normal babies every day in the United States. The danger arises when the virus is *not* dormant, and is being shed at the time of birth. Although a vulvar recurrence during pregnancy may not tend to affect the outcome of birth significantly, *severe* herpes cervicitis increases the risks of premature labor or of spontaneous abortion.

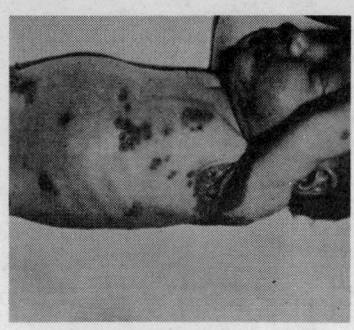
Neonatal herpes.
Herpes of Newborn.
Skin rash in infant
age 12 hours.

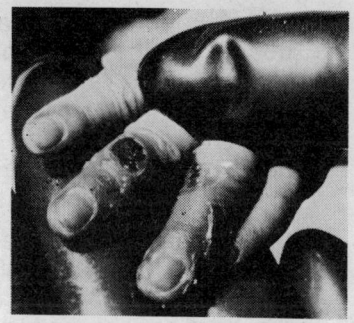
Ulcerative lesion
of finger. Same subject.

When genital lesions are present at the time of delivery, 25 to 45 percent of newborns will be infected. Such infection of the newborn medically is called neonatal herpes. Sometimes the baby is infected only locally. This kind of infection is neither too serious nor is it life-endangering, and the baby recovers completely. However, more often the disease becomes disseminated throughout the baby's body. Such a widespread dissemination produces a life-threatening infection. Of the infants who acquire herpes at the time of birth, 75 to 80 percent do not survive. At least 50% of those who do recover suffer from crippling abnormalities, the two most common of which are blindness and brain damage.

The chances of the baby becoming infected rise dramatically when the mother's membranes (bag of waters) have been ruptured for a substantial period of time — more than four to six hours preceding delivery. Open membranes enable the virus in and around the vagina to ascend and contaminate the baby. The virus attacks the baby through the nose, eyes, mouth or any opening or break in the skin. More than half the infants infected with herpes develop a massive infection, with the virus spreading to the blood (viremia) and consequently spreading through the body. The immune defense system of a newborn is immature. Having had no prior experience, the infant's defense mechanisms are unprepared to repel or resist the invading virus. For this reason such initial infection in infants are overwhelming. This accounts for the remarkably high fatality rate and for the similarly high rate of serious residual damage in survivors. The particular type of herpes simplex involved is of no consequence. While from 25 to 35 percent of all neonatal herpes cases are HSV-1 infections, the statistical outcome is the same as when the infection is HSV-2.

Diagnosing the disease in a newborn infant is facilitated greatly — and ironically enough — by the presence of herpetic lesions on the newborn's skin, mouth or eyes. In the absence of visible lesions, diagnosis often is not made early enough to be of much help to the child.

A high level of suspicion is required on the physician's part when dealing with a sick baby whose mother or whose mother's sexual partner(s) is known to have contracted herpes — especially, but not only, if the infection was that of genital herpes.

91. Is the risk to the infant greater if the mother has a primary infection of herpes or if the mother is experiencing a recurrence of herpes at term?

As noted, the immune defense system of an infant is immature and can not ward off infection. It is not until the infant is about two weeks old that its immune system has developed sufficiently to protect the infant from being ravaged by what otherwise would be a self-limited infestation. When a virus is present during pregnancy, the only protection an infant can receive, if it is exposed to the virus, comes from whatever antibodies are circulating within the mother's system. The mother's circulating antibodies can cross the placenta and be absorbed by the unborn child's own system.

Should the mother contract a primary infection while pregnant, there will be no circulating antibodies in her system for her to pass along to the fetus. The body manufactures viral antibodies only in response to infection, not in advance of or in anticipation of a viral infection. Thus the risk to the infant is greater if the mother has a primary infection of herpes. The risk to the infant is greatest when the mother's primary infection occurs within ten days of delivery. The mother's defense system is unable to manufacture a sufficient quantity of antibodies within that period of time for any significant, beneficial transfer of antibodies to the fetus.

The earlier during term the mother experiences a primary infection of herpes, the more time her body has to manufacture antibodies against the virus. In turn, the greater the quantity of antibodies which will cross the placenta, be absorbed by the fetus and so provide the infant with at least some degree of protection from the infection.

We know that recurrent attacks of herpes tend to be less severe, less frequent and of shorter duration. Thus the risk to the infant is less should the mother experience a recurrent attack than it would be were the attack a primary one. By the same token, the risk to the infant is diminished even further if the recurrent attack is the mother's tenth rather than her first. The fetus can not manufacture its own antibodies. It is dependent entirely upon receiving antibodies passively — that is, from the mother. Therefore, the more antibodies circulating within the mother's body, and the more efficient the mother's defense system is at manufacturing antibodies, the greater the protection offered the infant.

Also, because initial attacks are associated with a greater production of viral particles and the virus is usually shed for longer periods of time, the risk to the infants of mothers with primary herpes poses a greater threat than does recurrent disease. A problem arises, however, for despite the differences in the degree of risk it is not always easy for the physician to determine whether an infection of herpes in the mother is a primary or recurrent attack. Yet, it is unlikely the infant will contract herpes while within the uterus unless its mother has viremia — virus particles in the bloodstream. With viremia, the virus particles can enter the amniotic fluid, infecting the unborn fetus. While the physician may not be able to differentiate between a primary and a recurrent attack, he can detect the presence of virus in the amniotic fluid. And, viremia and in utero infection is most unusual in a recurrence. Almost invariably, viremia is a condition which accompanies primary herpes outbreaks.

92. What can be done to prevent congenital herpes?

If a pregnant woman or her sexual partner has or has had genital herpes, she should inform her doctor. Once informed, the physician can monitor for the presence of herpes throughout the pregnancy, and plan the best care for mother and baby. Many babies with congenital herpes are born to women with no symptoms of herpes. It is important to remember that infection in a partner may lead to congenital herpes even when the mother has never had any symptoms of the disease.

93. What factors play a role in deciding whether to perform special lab tests and to consider doing a caesarean section at the time of delivery?

The decision of whether or not to perform a caesarean section is based upon the relative benefits the procedure offers for mother and infant. If there is any question whatsoever about active disease and viral shedding by the mother when she is at term — ready to deliver — the risk of infection to the infant makes caesarean section the delivery procedure of choice. If the mother is experiencing a primary infection of herpes at term, then a caesarean section is mandatory. The sole exception to this would be if the woman's bag of waters had been ruptured from four to six hours because the virus would have had sufficient time to ascend to the uterus. Under these circumstances an expeditious vaginal delivery would be preferable.

94. How many smears or cultures should be taken near term to determine if the virus is active and being shed?

Again, this depends upon the woman's prior history of herpes infection and the currently perceived possible risks of the infant contracting the disease. Such criteria vary greatly from person to person. Of particular importance is that the mother-to-be report immediately to her doctor any prodromal symptoms, recurrences or lesions developing at new, previously uninfested sites.

Screening with viral cultures should be instituted between 30 and 36 weeks following conception. This should leave about a month, give or take, before delivery. Viral cultures are the most reliable of the basic tests, yet require up to two days before results are available. As delivery becomes imminent, a test yielding faster results may be required. Thus toward the end of term a series of pap smears may be performed. While the pap smear is not as sensitive as is the viral culture, its results are obtained in a matter of hours. Repeated testing is helpful in the detection of silent shedding.

If the expectant mother lives near one of the larger university centers, she may be able to avail herself of electron microscopy. The results from this form of testing are highly accurate and are obtained almost immediately.

Women with no lesions, no evidence of viral shedding and negative pap smears and viral cultures are good candidates for normal, vaginal delivery.

95. Will delivery by caesarean section while the membranes are still intact guarantee the baby will not have herpes?

There are few, if any, guarantees in medicine. Rarely, caesarean section will fail to protect the newborn even though the membranes are intact. The notable exception is the rare instance when the mother experiences a viremia — virus in the bloodstream. This rare situation is most often encountered when the mother is experiencing her primary attack during pregnancy. When viremia is present, the viral infection crosses the placenta and contaminates the amniotic fluid in which the fetus lives. It is possible, through a procedure called amniocentesis, to examine the amniotic fluid for the presence of herpes. This test, in conjunction with a viral culture, is very reliable.

Should the test be positive, no advantages will be reaped from performing a caesarean section, since infection of the infant would have already occurred.

96. Can a newborn contract herpes postpartum even if its mother does not have genital herpes?

Yes. Such cases are far less common than those acquired from the mother's infected birth canal; however, the consequences to the infant are the same. Recent studies have proved *some* cases to be a result of herpes labialis, the plain old herpes of the lips: fever blister. It is estimated that up to 24% of adults with active herpes labialis of the HSV-1 strain normally shed the virus without displaying any symptoms whatsoever of the virus's activity. Further studies have shown the herpes virus, when mixed with saliva, as it is in instances of herpes of the lips, can be shed in droplet form when speaking or even during respiration. Also, in saliva-droplet form, the virus can survive on skin, on cloth (garments, sheets, blankets, etc.) and on plastic for some time. Thus, one could expect to find the herpes virus on the hands of persons with herpes labialis infections (many persons invariably touch their mouths regularly), without the concurrent presence of herpes whitlow being necessary.

Individuals with a herpes infection, as characterized above, can be found almost anywhere, including at work in a pediatric nursery in a hospital. And, a silently shed virus can be transmitted to a newborn as easily as can a viral infection accompanied by visible symptoms. So, the threat to the infant of exposure to herpes contraction of the disease is quite real.

While definitive proof of such contamination contributing to the number of cases of deadly neonatal herpes is lacking, very strong circumstantial evidence certainly does exist to support such a conclusion. Closely related to the preceding is whether a newborn should be isolated from its mother if she has a herpes fever blister. As difficult and possibly traumatic (primarily for the mother) as such a measure would be, mothers with active herpes lesions on their skin should at least keep them covered. Remember, physical stress is a potent triggering mechanism for the reactivation of the herpes virus, and childbearing certainly has many physically stressful qualities to it.

The post-natal danger comes to the baby in the form of being kissed or fondled. Kissing can spread the virus directly to the mucous membranes of the baby's nose, mouth or eyes. Furthermore, as most persons know, small infants incessantly stretch and touch, and derive pleasure from placing their hands in their mouths. The potential this poses for the infant's contraction of the virus is obvious, especially when the infant has touched its mother's mouth or lips: something an infant commonly does. Friends and relatives known to have herpes should be kept away from newborns. By the time the baby reaches one month of age, its immune system will have developed sufficiently that the disease no longer poses the same serious life-threatening danger it did during the first few weeks of life.

The possibility of the newborn contracting herpes while in the nursery being known, any newborn in whom herpes is suspected should be isolated from the other infants in the nursery. A baby need not contract the disease from an adult; any human carrier, including another baby, can transmit the virus.

To place the question of postpartum contraction of herpes in perspective, it must be noted the theoretical possibilities by far outdistance the practical ones. Indeed, if one dwells upon the theoretical possibilities of postpartum infection, the imagination can run rampant and wild and become positively staggered. Because they do exist, and because postpartum infection does occur, these possibilities have been discussed. However, with reasonable, common sense precautionary care, the practical possibilities of the postpartum contraction of herpes by the infant can be minimized to an acceptable level, posing no special threat.

PART VII:
Herpes and Cancer

97. What is the relationship between herpes and cancer?

Some viruses of the herpes family have been shown to cause cancer in laboratory animals. Such findings make *all* the herpes viruses suspect, even though most of these suspicions can neither be confirmed nor denied. Questions researchers now are attempting to answer are: Are the viruses themselves the culprits? Or, are the viruses associates of the culprits? Or, are segments from the viruses' DNA the causative agent? Or, do the viruses merely drive the "get-away car", so to speak? The answers to these questions can not all be "no". By the same token, they can not all be "yes", either.

Women with cervical herpes have at least a three- to fivefold greater incidence of cervical cancer than women without cervical herpes. Conversely, women with cervical cancer have a high incidence of elevated antibody titers to the herpes simplex viruses.

Accordingly, women with herpes are advised to have a pap smear at least once a year; twice a year would be ideal. While an annual pap smear almost always will detect cervical cancer in an early enough stage to cure it, a semi-annual test removes the word "almost" — a word well worth removing from the statement. The evolutionary cycle through which cells go as they change from normal to pre-cancerous to cancerous is a lengthy cycle. Regular pap smears are a good preventive measure, and thus a habit all women, *especially* those who have experienced an outbreak of cervical herpes, should cultivate.

Fortunately, the overall rate of cervical cancer is low. Also fortunately, the cervix is a site at which monitoring (with the pap smear) is accomplished easily. With semi-annual monitoring of the cervix, and with the prompt initiation of appropriate treatment if pre-cancerous cellular changes are noted, the cure rate is — again most fortunately — almost perfect.

An increased incidence of vulvar cancer definitely has been noted in women with genital herpes. However, vulvar cancer can be detected readily, because it develops slowly and is superficial. Being superficial, it can be seen easily. The lesions may be raised, and their coloring may be that of normal skin, whitish, grey or pigmented. While the vast majority of skin lesions in the vulvar area is benign and unrelated to herpes infection, any growths, bumps or sections of raised skin a woman may notice demand medical evaluation by her physician.

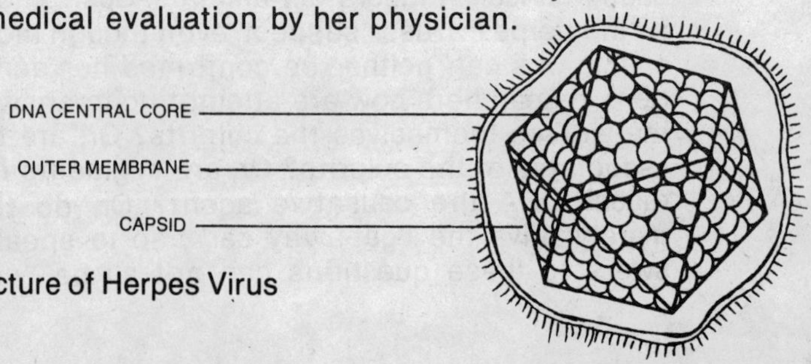

Fig. 8 – Structure of Herpes Virus

PART VIII:
The Life Cycle of the Herpes Virus and Body Defenses

98. What is a virus?

A virus is a non-cellular parasite so is only able to reproduce inside a living cell. The living cell a virus invades is called the host cell. A host organism is any living entity, such as a person, that has been invaded by a parasite, such as the herpes virus.

The chemical structure of the herpes virus consists of a core composed of nucleic acid — DNA (deoxyribonucleic Acid). DNA is the same chemical substance of which human chromosomes are made. Surrounding this central core of genetic material is an outer coating of protein called the *capsid.* The herpes viruses also have an outer fatty membrane which is like an envelope for the virus and is quite similar to the membrane which covers the host cell from which it is derived (Fig. 8).

As complex as a virus is, it nevertheless is a *relatively* simple chemical substance when compared with the many chemicals, and the bio-chemical and physical interactions and balances in which a living cell engages in the processes that constitute what is called "life".

Some viruses, like most chemicals, can be synthesized in the laboratory. Some viruses, too, like an ordinary chemical, can be crystallized, and thus stored on a shelf indefinitely without losing any of their ability to reproduce themselves when inside their respective appropriate host cells.

Viruses are smaller than are bacteria, and, unlike bacteria, can not be seen when using an ordinary microscope. They are visible, though, with the tremendous magnification generated by the electron microscope. The electron microscope directs a beam of electrons instead of light at the object being examined. A "shadow" of the object forms the image which is viewed.

Viruses are measured in units called nanometers (nm). One nanometer is 1/1,000,000,000th or 0.000000001 of a meter. One inch contains about 25 million nanometers. The herpes simplex virus measures about 150 nanometers. To span an entire inch, 165,000 herpes simplex virus particles would have to be laid end-to-end.

It is difficult to appreciate such small sizes. When viewed through an ordinary microscope, under a 1,000 power magnification, an ordinary red blood cell appears to have a diameter of about one-eighth of an inch. The white blood cells are even larger than are the red ones (Fig. 9). When viewed under an electron microscope, the same red blood cell which actually only measures 7,500 nanometers in diameter appears quite large. Thus the size of various viruses, including the herpes simplex, can be seen in contrast with the circumference of the red blood cell as shown in Figure 10. Rather like craters on the moon!

An individual viral particle is called a virion. The herpes virion does have a precise physical structure, called an icosahedron. Geometrically, an icosahedron has 20 triangular surfaces, 30 edges and 12 corners (Fig. 11).

While all viruses certainly are organic substances, there is no agreement as to whether or not they are living organisms. Many definitions of life have been proferred, but none have been accepted universally. The characteristics and behavior of viruses lie in the grey areas of the possible definitions of "Is this a living thing?"

Everyone knows for sure a dog is alive and a rock is not. Every living organism has boundaries between it and its environment. A living organism, for instance, can reproduce itself and can obtain energy from chemicals it absorbs from its environment. A virus can not do this. It can not transform energy for reproductive or for any other purposes. Viruses can not respond to their environments. As noted, they lack cellular organization. Yet, while viruses lack many of the chemicals of life, they certainly are unique if they are non-living. If viruses are alive, they just as certainly are the smallest, most basic organism known to exist.

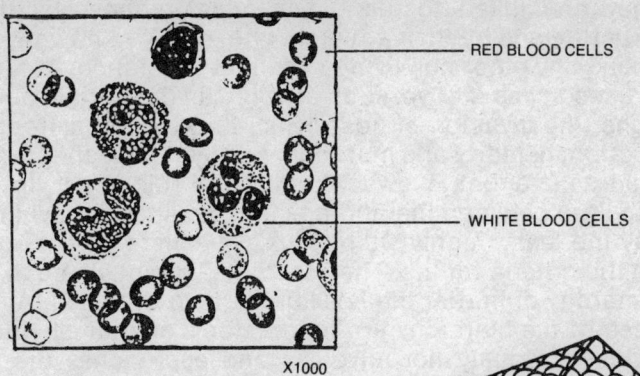

Fig. 9 – Blood Cells

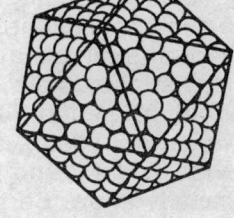

Fig. 11 – Icosahederal Shape of the Herpes Virus

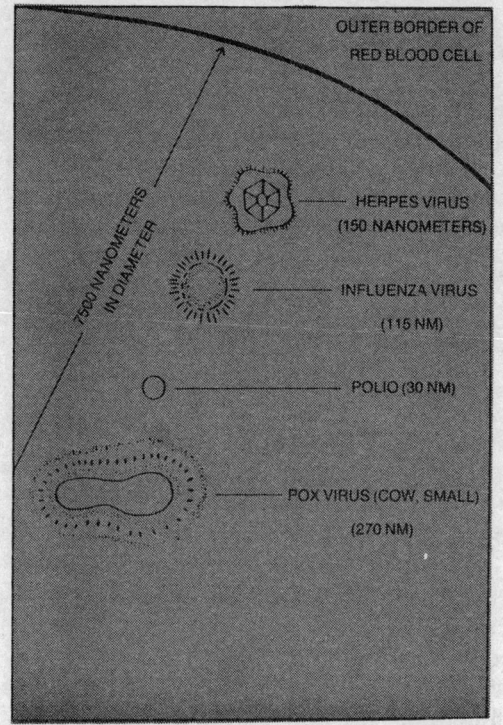

Fig. 10 – Comparison of Size of Herpes Virus with Red Blood Cell

They are linked to the bio-chemical process by their structure and by their apparent "life cycle". And, they are unlike any other non-living chemical substance. At times viruses act as if alive, such as when, under certain conditions (the invasion of host cells), they exhibit self-reproduction, heredity and mutation. At other times they are as inert as is a rock. Viewed literally, it would seem viruses vacillate between life and non-life; yet such a view is, to say the least, highly suspicious. Scientists do not agree on the criteria for life. They can not pinpoint where in the hierarchy of matter the level of life is to be found. At the base of the hierarchy are found atoms and simple molecules, obviously not alive. As one approaches the top nucleic acids are encountered. And finally, upon reaching the pinnacle one finds the very complicated and sophisticated, and obviously alive, cellular substances. A definition that does no more than confirm the obvious is not very useful, and the working definitions we have of life so far do no more than that: they tell us what we already know. Be that as it may, it *is* known just what viruses can and will do and just what they can not and will not do. Until subsequent refinements in scientific enquiry enable the more subtle questions about the nature of the virus to be answered, one must regard such distinctions and questions as being those of semantics and focus upon what is known, and by being known, useful.

Viruses cause a wide variety of diseases other than herpes. The common cold, measles, mumps, polio, rabies and hepatitis are but a few of the great number of viral diseases known.

99. What is the natural life cycle of the herpes virus?

First, the virus attaches itself to receptors located on the surface of a host cell. After affixing itself to the receptors the virus' outer member fuses with the host's cell membrane. The virus then sheds its envelope and enters the host cell. The invaded cell, although it dooms itself in the process, secretes an enzyme substance which strips the virus of its capsid covering. The released DNA central core of the virus is now propelled to the nucleus of the host cell where cellular take-over commences. The viral DNA commandeers the nuclear machinery of the host cell which is then put to work replicating viral DNA. At the same time the host cell creates new protein coverings (capsids) for the newly manufactured viral DNA. The new capsid is then merged with the viral DNA. The completion of this union marks the birth of another virus (Fig. 12).

The new virus can pass from its host cell through adjoining cell walls and attack neighboring host cells without entering the extracellular spaces — the lymph or bloodstream. The virus thus avoids contact with antibodies and defensive host cells which circulate there, ever ready to neutralize viral invaders (Fig. 13).

Another route of spread sometimes utilized by the herpes virus involves the rupturing of the host cell after it becomes distended with many thousands of viral particles. To become infectious when liberated by this route, the virus must first acquire its outer envelope. It is as it leaves the host cell that the new virus appropriates a segment of the host cell membrane as its own outer covering. Now it may attack other cells (Fig. 14). Viral attack is random and undirected. Viruses spread by attacking any susceptible cell with which they chance to come in contact, usually cells close by. The 25,000 to 80,000 herpes virus particles the infected host cell can produce is a process taking from four to five hours. Each liberated viral particle, in turn, will seek to attach itself to the outer wall receptors of available host cells. Here the entire cycle will begin anew. As more host cells are invaded — that is, as the virus spreads, the individual begins to experience the early symptoms of herpes. If the infection is not promptly controlled he soon develops the painful lesion caused by the viral invader.

Sometimes the herpes virus invades the host cell, sets up housekeeping and replicates in harmony with its host without disrupting the host cell's vital cellular processes. This *steady state* mutual living arrangement between virus and host explains those cases of silent viral shedding in the completely asymptomatic individual.

100. How does the body protect itself from the onslaught of the herpes virus?

Upon encountering the virus, the susceptible host has a

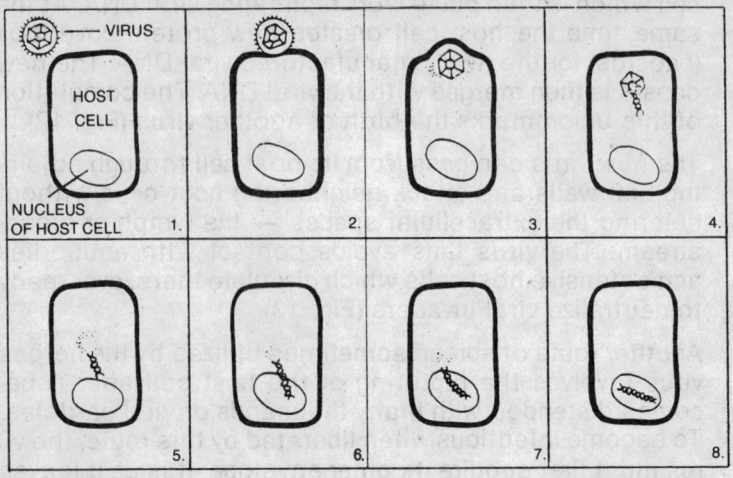

1. VIRUS APPROACHES HOST CELL.
2. VIRUS AFFIXES TO HOST CELL.
3. VIRUS ENTERS HOST CELL.
4. OUTER COATING OF VIRUS BEGINS TO DESOLVE, EXPOSING DNA CORE.
5.-7. DNA PROPELLED TO HOST CELL NUCLEUS, WHICH IT PENETRATES.
8. PENETRATION COMPLETE, CELL TAKEOVER BEGINS.

Fig. 12 – Natural Life Cycle of Herpes Virus

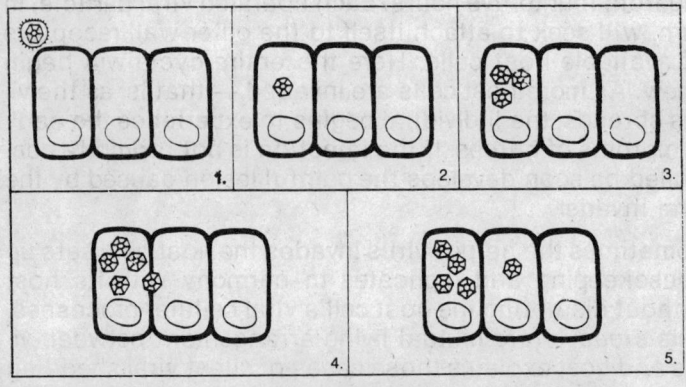

1. VIRUS APPROACHES HOST CELL
2. VIRUS PENETRATES AND ENTERS HOST CELL
3. VIRUS REPLICATES IN HOST CELL
4. VIRUS BEGINS TO CROSS CELL MEMBRANE AND ENTER ADJOINING HOST CELL
5. CYCLE REPEATS

Fig. 13 – Cell to Cell Route of Viral Spread

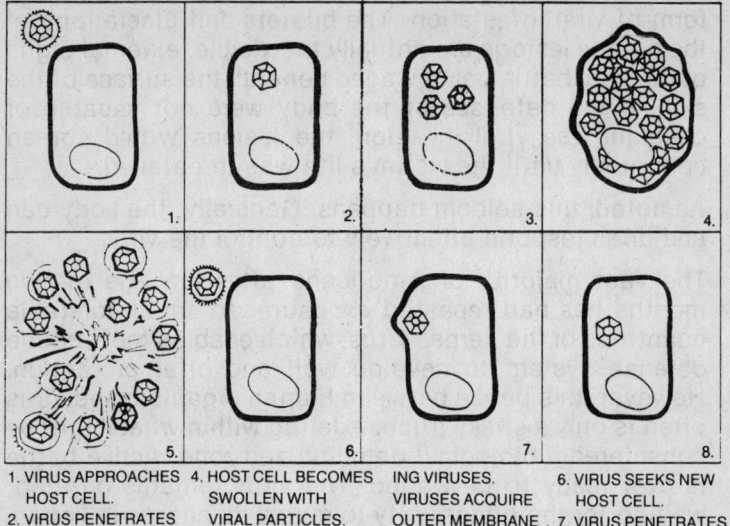

1. VIRUS APPROACHES HOST CELL.
2. VIRUS PENETRATES HOST CELL.
3. VIRUS REPLICATES
4. HOST CELL BECOMES SWOLLEN WITH VIRAL PARTICLES.
5. HOST CELL EXPLODES, LIBERATING VIRUSES. VIRUSES ACQUIRE OUTER MEMBRANE AS THEY LEAVE HOST CELL.
6. VIRUS SEEKS NEW HOST CELL.
7. VIRUS PENETRATES NEW HOST CELL.
8. CYCLE REPEATS.

Fig. 14 – Viral Spread (Cont.)

number of specific and non-specific defense mechanisms at its disposal. The non-specific mechanisms are the general forms of protection always on hand which work against invasion broadly, rather than specifically against the particular viral invader.

The body's first line of defense is a simple mechanical barrier: the intact skin or mucous membrane. Obviously, in the absence of physical entrance, viral penetration can not occur. Additionally, secretions from the skin and mucous surfaces can have antiviral properties.

When these first line defensive techniques succeed, infection is prevented. When they fail, infection occurs, usually by the virus establishing a localized foot-hold. Rarely, the virus goes on to gain entry into the bloodstream. It then becomes disseminated throughout the body, and can seed multiple distal sites of infection. This form of viral infection scarcely happens. When it does, it is most likely to occur to infants under about two weeks of age and to those whose immune system have been compromised.

The localized herpes lesion is the typical, garden-variety form of viral infestation. The blisters and ulcerations of the herpes lesions are actually the visible, external signs of the viral battle being waged beneath the surface of the skin. If the defenses of the body were not capable of checking the viral invasion, the lesions would spread continually until the victim's life was threatened.

As noted, this seldom happens. Generally, the body can and does respond effectively to control the virus.

The vast majority of Americans after the age of two months has had repeated exposures to small, tolerable quantities of the herpes virus, which enables the immune defense system to develop well and offer protection. However, this peace between human organism and virus often is only a shaky truce, existing within what might be considered a biological demilitarized zone. Active battle is ever ready to be waged. The virus remains on alert, waiting for the opportunity to renew its charge in yet another attempt to subdue the carrier host.

The way in which the host cells successfully repel a viral attack involves an extremely complex series of actions, reactions and inter-actions among cells and sub-cellular and bio-chemical components of the body. All work is in concert to respond to the foreign substance within — the herpes virus. What follows is a simplified sequence of events, which will help the reader understand the general nature of the battle waged between body and virus.

The hallmark of an efficient immune defense system is the ability to distinguish between normal, healthy cells and infected cells. After the host cell has been invaded by the virus, and as the host cell's normal biological functions cease, the cellular wall of the host cell undergoes modification. The changes which occur alert the immune defense system to the presence of the virus. It is as though the host cell hoists a banner proclaiming its state of siege. This makes the infected host cell an easily identifiable target for the body's defensive army, the immune defense system. This army-of-sorts has two main divisions: (1) humoral immunity, the type associated with the production of antibodies; and (2) cell-mediated. It is the job of the cellular elements to seek out and destroy the invaders. One element of the cellular army, the macrophages, accumulate in large numbers on the viral battlefield. These cells devour cellular, viral and biochemical debris. Such debris exists in large quantities due to the lethal attacks of other special units of the cellular army, which kill infected host cells which contain viruses. The key to controlling the spread of the virus is the self-regulated destruction of infected cells by the internal resources of the host organism.

When a viral battle results in a victory for the host organism, no further banners proclaiming infestation are hoisted. The infected cells and their invaders have been eradicated. Therefore, a reason to proclaim infestation of the host organism no longer exists. The batallions of host killer cells return to their barracks — their resting places in the lymph nodes and bone marrow. The antibody-producing cells likewise withdraw. The macrophages clean up any last, remaining debris and then return to the bone marrow, from where they were first summoned.

The push and pull between virus and host ends. When this occurs, the infection abates and the virus becomes dormant. Tissue regeneration commences. In a matter of days, the fields of viral battle — which are, of course, the herpes lesions — have healed. The virus will remain dormant until some fresh condition — not the least of which is mental stress — triggers reactivation of the virus. When stimulated by such a fresh insult, another viral battle will brew and soon thereafter will be fought.

The veterans of the viral battle — the host's defensive army — and many, many other constituents of the immune defense system — remember their encounters with the virus, and actually learn from those encounters. What they learn is the enemy code — the unique markings of the herpes virus. When next summoned, even upon short notice, these veterans are better prepared than they previously were to engage the virus in combat. They will respond more rapidly and more adeptly in the future and will have less difficulty in containing the virus. In other words, the host organism has developed an acquired immunity. This immunity will serve the host well into future, perhaps for life, and explains why recurrent attacks of the virus tend to decrease in severity, in frequency and in duration. However, as medical resources exist today, numerous battles — but never the war — can be won.

PART IX:
The Sociological Aspects of Herpes

101. What is the most important sociological step toward combatting herpes?

The best initial step toward combatting genital herpes is to dispel the social stigma attached to the disease, for this stigma is the major impediment of genuine knowledge and understanding. Such knowledge and understanding, coupled with what treatments there are to reduce the severity of and the complications from attacks of genital herpes, are the keystones to dealing succesfully with herpes.

102. Has public thinking about herpes changed in the past few years?

It has indeed, and dramatically. The surge in genital herpes is relatively recent, and the current epidemic level has had a significant impact. The sexual revolution of the 1960's led to increased sexual freedom and with it rose the opportunity for transmitting herpes. Now, possibly contracting such an unpleasant disorder is putting a damper on sexual freedom.

103. Has the media caused fears about herpes to be blown out of proportion?

News is often sensationalized and the medical community is in agreement that this was the case with herpes. Fortunately, the promotion of misleading information regarding this common virus gradually diminished. Physicians, health educators and the medical community at large have united to combat the spread of both herpes and the myths which surround it. Once unnecessary fear is overcome by knowledge of the facts regarding herpes, victims will be able to control the disease and the number of potential sufferers should decline. Hopefully, the media will assist the efforts of the medical community to properly educate the public about herpes.

104. Has herpes affected attitudes toward sexual activity?

The herpes scare generated by the media initially caused national fear of contracting an "incurable" disease. Fortunately, factual education of the public regarding prevention and control of herpes is clearing up the many myths about this disorder and may eventually reduce both the incidence and unnecessary phobias surrounding this virus.

105. How has herpes affected attitudes toward the "one night stand"?

Due to the marked increase in genital herpes cases, the old "one night stand" has new implications. Herpes lasts forever — passion may only last for a moment. Since the most common source of transmission for herpes is during indiscriminate sexual activity without use of precautionary measures, public attitude toward the "one night stand" has become less liberal.

Regardless of what moral judgments some persons feel compelled to make, and whether or not such judgments are correct or incorrect, the simple fact of the matter is that what commonly is called promiscuity immeasurably enhances one's chances of contracting herpes.

106. Do prostitutes have a high incidence of herpes infections?

Certain recent studies among groups of prostitutes revealed the rate of infection to be as high as it could be: 100%. Prostitution, of course, is the most graphic embodiment of the "one night stand" attitude. Even though less mercantile embodiments no doubt result in less high rates of infection, the tendency is obvious.

107. Has herpes been affected by changes in birth control techniques?

Prior to the introduction of "The Pill", the frequency of sexual encounters for women was curtailed due to fears of pregnancy. In combination with the sexual freedom advocated in the 1960s, "The Pill" undoubtedly has contributed to the spread of herpes.

The decline in popularity of the condom — an excellent mechanical barrier — and the diaphragm and spermicidal jellies has also contributed to the spread of the disease.

The ability of the herpes virus to recur is still the single most important reason for the continued increase in cases. The virus is spread logarithmically. Each new case is spread to two others who in turn infect two others. The following three factors also have had significant effects on the incidence of herpes:
1. more individuals are having sex — at younger and older ages
2. more often and with
3. a greater number of partners.

108. Do many people overreact to herpes?

Admittedly, herpes victims suffer, and no form of suffering is pleasant to endure, yet this is not the aspect of genital herpes to which over-reaction is probable. Over-reaction to genital herpes is seen in the way a person alters his perception of himself, especially his self-esteem. And this, too, is one way in which our thinking about herpes has changed in recent years.

Many people regard genital herpes as *some* form of punishment ministered by *some* superior presence for having done *something* bad or wrong. In other words, genital herpes generates a lot of guilt, and people flagellate themselves mentally for having contracted it. Occasionally, people regard themselves as akin to lepers. Such thinking is completely unwarranted, and the recognition of this is one of the fortunate ways in which our thinking about herpes has changed for the better.

People regularly catch colds and other, minor maladies from each other while engaged in mutal expressions of sexual affection. There being nothing bad or wrong about such sexual exchanges, the mode of transmission being exactly the same (i.e. sexual activity) regardless of the malady transmitted and neither party making a deliberate attempt to contract or to transmit any malady, it becomes clear the reaction to *having contracted* herpes should be neither more nor less than the reaction to having contracted, for instance, a cold or the flu. The reaction to *having* herpes well may differ from the reaction to having a cold or the flu, because here a legitimate difference exists: herpes is neither a cold nor the flu. And yet, as has been stated, herpes per se is exceptionally common.

Without doubt, we must differentiate between the disease itself and the fact the disease can manifest itself visibly in the genital area. Having drawn this distinction clearly is having taken a giant stride forward.

PART X:
Herpes Resources

109. Is there a resource that provides on-going information and counseling for individuals with herpes?

Yes. The American Social Health Association, a national, non-profit health foundation, sponsors a membership designed to assist herpes sufferers. The program, called the Herpes Resource Center (formerly HELP), provides members with a quarterly newsletter (*The HELPER*), operates a telephone hotline, and organizes local self-help groups. For more information, send a stamped, self-addressed envelope to ASHA, P.O. Box 100, Palo Alto, California 94302.

The VD National Hotline can provide additional information on herpes and other sexually transmitted diseases. The toll-free number *except* in California is, 1-800-227-8922; in California, the telephone number (also toll-free) is 1-800-982-5883.

Look in the classified section of your newspaper for announcements on local meetings for herpes sufferers. Or call the out-patient department of a local hospital for referrals to herpes counseling clinics and support groups.

PART XI:
AIDS

110. Does the homosexual community have a higher incidence of herpes, STD's in general, or a related problem?

STD's are on the rise in the homosexual community but there *is* a problem far more severe than the STD's including herpes, with which the male homosexual community is contending. The problem is infectious in nature, possibly related to a virus which is like a "country cousin" to the herpes virus. This virus cytomegalovirus (CMV) is common and usually causes nothing more than symptoms similar to that of a common cold.

However, under certain conditions, herpes "country cousin" can turn mean: CMV can cause "immunosuppression", interfering with the body's ability to fight off infections and invasions from bacteria, viruses, even cancer, although the degree of immunosuppression caused by CMV *usually* is not severe.

111. What is Kaposi's sarcoma?

Kaposi's sarcoma (pronounced ka-POH-shee's sar-KOH-ma) is one form of cancer to which the immunosuppressed individual is highly susceptible.* This cancer causes tumors on the skin and mucous membranes. Until 1981, it was a very rare disease and attacks were isolated and mild. The medical community now treats a significantly increased number of cases which are aggressive and can be lethal, usually affecting homosexual males. The cytomegalovirus has been cultured successfully from 40% of cases of Kaposi's sarcoma.

> *Note:* Kaposi's sarcoma has also been reported in those who inject drugs, or products from pooled blood, and in recipients of multiple blood transfusions.

Kaposi's cancer is most common in the sexually active homosexual male. It is far more prevalent in male homosexuals than in male heterosexuals, in males than in females, and in females married to bisexual males than in females married to heterosexual males.

112. Is Kaposi's sarcoma related to AIDS?

AIDS is an acronym for "Acquired Immune Deficiency Syndrome". AIDS is not a single disease, but a group of symptoms related to reduced immunosuppression. Kaposi's sarcoma is considered to be one of the "marker" illnesses of AIDS (since it is rearely seen in young individuals unless AIDS is present).

113. What causes AIDS?

AIDS does not have a single known specific cause. The illnesses associated with AIDS are cuased by various infections which take advantage of a vulnerable (i.e. immunosuppressed) body. Usually, the body can defend itself against most of the viruses, bacteria and other organisms which exist in the environment, but when the immune system is weakened by AIDS, the normal defense is lowered.

114. Does overwork cause the body's immune defense system to break down?

In Haiti, parasitic infestation has been rampant for years and years, yet AIDS is a new phenomenon. This finding has discredited the theory that suggested the repeated onslaught of infectious diseases that a disproportionate number of male homosexuals do contract made additional demands upon their immune defense systems. In turn, their system eventually decompensated, or broke down. No doubt such a theory would have been very useful had it been proven true, but it just doesn't make physiological sense. The immune defense system is quite resilient, and just does not break down in the face of an extra-heavy work load

115. What are the symptoms of AIDS?

The earliest symptoms are loss of appetite and fatigue. Patches of white — a fungus infection — may appear in the mouth. Fever may be present, body temperature soaring as high as 103°F. Night sweats are common, lymph glands swell, and diarrhea may occur. A series of recurring viral infections such as colds and flus, as well as herpes, is frequently observed. As AIDS continues to progress, pneumonia may occur and Kaposi's sarcoma become apparent in about one-third of the cases.

116. Is Kaposi's sarcoma the only type of malignancy associated wtih AIDS?

Initially, the tumors associated with AIDS were all Kaposi's sarcoma. Now a variety of other malignancies is being encountered. Most commonly reported have been a kind of lymph gland tumor called non-Hodgkin's lymphoma. Also reported have been squamous cell cancers of the tongue and of the rectum. The lymphomas have been exceptionally deadly. The tumor cells are of the type abbreviated DUNHL, which stands for diffuse, undifferentiated, non-Hodgkin's lymphoma. Several of these cases appeared microscopically to be *Burkitt's Lymphoma,* a type of malignancy seen in connection with the Epstein-Barr herpes virus. The Epstein-Barr is the strain which causes infectious mononucleosis; and under certain conditions, "mono" is associated with this type of tumor.

117. Is AIDS a new disorder?

AIDS has only been recognized for a short time. It was in April of 1981 when reports were first received of young male homosexuals from New York City who were dying of illnesses previously found in only markedly debilitated or immunosuppressed individuals.

It was first believed that AIDS was spread to the U.S. from Haiti, as a number of cases were noted in Haitian immigrants. However, scientists discovered that AIDS was first recognized in Haiti at the same time it was discovered in the U.S. and is no longer believed to have come to America from this small island.

In June, 1981, Florida physicians were asked to report

cases of AIDS in that state and followed by the establishment of a national task force to investigate the disorder. Currently, three cases per day are reported in the U.S. From the time of AIDS recognition until the present, there have been some 1,400 reported incidences, but there may be many more undiagnosed or misdiagnosed cases.

No one knows where or how AIDS began. And no one knows who will next be victimized by AIDS. AIDS is beginning to spread to the population at large, although it is still found primarily in male homosexuals.*

Although there is no hard scientific data, one theory purports AIDS to be related to AFRICAN SWINE fever. Although thought to be harmless to humans, this big viral illness bears certain superficial similarities to AIDS. Infected animals develop purplish skin lesions, run a fever, exhibit lymph node enlargement and generally run a progressive and fatal downhill course.

> *Note:* The only segment of the adult population which is relatively unaffected by AIDS is the female homosexual group. Lesbians have an exceedingly low rate of STD's which favors the theory that AIDS is sexually transmitted.

118. How contagious is AIDS?

There is no universal agreement among experts about how contagious it is. Professional medical personnel who work closely with AIDS victims have not been shown to be at risk candidates for developing AIDS. The disease does not seem to be spread by an airborne vehicle. Being in the same room with AIDS victims, using the same toilet facilities or eating at the same table with them does not seem to pose any hazard.

What does seem to be necessary to catch AIDS is intimate sexual contact, particularly activities permitting the sharing of blood, such as the minute abrasions which occur during anal intercourse. The blood, semen or saliva and possibly sweat from an individual with AIDS must be considered infectious. Contact with these body fluids from an AIDS victim is both a possible and theoretical route of transference.

Blood sharing also occurs among injectible-drug users who do not employ disposable paraphernalia. Even the minute quantity of 1/100th of a cubic centimeter (cc) of blood remaining in a previously employed syringe or needle is sufficient to transmit hepatitis. Therefore, it likewise must be considered a serious potential source for AIDS transmissison.

Although health workers have not yet shown any increased incidence of the syndrome when working with AIDS patients more than when working with any other group of patients, it certainly is advisable to take precautions, as it is whenever one is in close proximity with any form of infection. Strict isolation techniques should be employed by health workers treating AIDS victims.

Recent cases of AIDS in infants strongly suggests the syndrome may be more contagious than was formerly thought. Current evidence, however, suggests that these cases are a result of infection by the baby while still in the uterus. AIDS is spreading at a faster rate than anyone dared to imagine when the syndrome was first diagnosed in 1981.

It has been suggested that the epidemiology of Hepatitis B, a viral disease affecting the liver, may be a possible model for the spread of AIDS. Both disorders strike the same sub-groups: homosexuals, Haitians, intravenous drug users, recipients of pooled whole blood products and recipients of individual units of blood, the latter to a lesser degree than those receiving products derived from the combination of elements derived from many blood units such as those used in the treatment of hemophilia. Type B hepatitis virus has been isolated not only from blood and lymph tissues but semen, saliva, sweat and mucus.

119. How is AIDS treated?

The basic defect that causes AIDS and paves the way for the associated Kaposi's sarcoma as yet has not been amenable to specific treatment. This basic defect is, of course, immunosuppression. The secondary manifestations of the syndrome — the infections which affect the vulnerable body — are treated, to the extent feasible, with antibiotics. Experimental treatments that have been tried include bone-marrow transplants, plasma exchange transfusions from healthy donors, Interferon and the injection of an experimental extract from immune defense cells called transfer factor. Thus far, results have been far from dramatic.

120. Is AIDS a fatal disorder?

Fewer than 14% of AIDS victims survive for more than three years after diagnosis is established. No known victim has ever fully recovered. The drugs used to treat the different infections may be initially successful, but are not capable of curing the succession of infections which occur.

121. How is AIDS diagnosed?

To make a diagnosis of AIDS physicians do not begin with the pathologist's benefit of hindsight. A clinician may be confronted by a patient who has an overwhelming encephalitis or pneumonia. Yet the clinician would have no reason to suspect other than an infestation from a particularly virulent organism. Accordingly, diagnosis is especially difficult in the earlier stages of the disorder. No specific diagnostic test for AIDS exists, since AIDS is really a syndrome, with numerous disorders as a reflection of the underlying immune deficiency. "Marker" illnesses include pneumonia and Kaposi's sarcoma, as well as encephalitis and herpes. When seen in conjunction with one another, a diagnosis of AIDS can be made.

122. Is there a good side to AIDS?

Many dark clouds do have silver linings. The relationship between AIDS and cancer could lead to a breakthrough in cancer research. A viral link to many cancers has been suspected for years and demonstrated in the laboratory. Thus, AIDS may be a key to understanding this link and controling it.

123. How can individuals who need blood transfusions protect themselves against AIDS?

If the need for surgery is known in advance, individuals can donate their own blood in advance. If that is not possible, it is best to use blood from volunteer donors. Paid donors are often alcoholic, may not reveal their past histories regarding infectious diseases, and may not practice good hygiene. Volunteer blood donors tend to be concerned with the consequences for the recipients.

124. What is the single, most important thing a male homosexual can do to avoid AIDS?

Limit sexual promiscuity. One steady relationship is the best insurance available. Contrary-wise, the single, most predisposing factor is frequent sexual relations with different partners.

125. Should all contact with male homosexuals be avoided to protect against AIDS?

Sexual contact should be avoided of course, and sharing of body secretions. This includes kissing, sharing toothbrushes or eating utensils, and trading razors. There is no need to avoid gays like the plague, however.

126. How important is hygiene in AIDS prevention?

The "at risk" groups all seem to share defects in hygiene. These defects may be either in general personal hygiene or in sexual practices that permit infectious body fluids to be shared. (It should be noted sexual activity is not particularly hygienic, per se.) Consider the Haitians, who have a disproportionate share of AIDS cases. Most exist at poverty level, where personal hygiene tends to be at its lowest. And, many male homosexuals have intimate sexual contact without very much regard for hygienic conditions.

127. Where can an individual call for further information on AIDS?

There is a toll-free crisis line maintained by the National Gay Task Force weekdays from 3:00 p.m. to 9:00 p.m. The number is 1-800-221-7044.

PART XII:
The Legal Aspects of Herpes

128. What are the lawsuits involving herpes that have received so much publicity recently all about?

This contemporary American society of ours is, to say the very least, entrenched firmly in the belief that the universal solution to all problems is litigation. Indeed, the bringing of civil actions perhaps is one of the few diseases rivalling or even surpassing herpes in incidence. No complaint is too slight or too frivolous to forestall redress through our (highly efficient) judicial system. Though the broader issues of this phenomenon would constitute a separate volume, far lengthier than this one, in itself, it should be noted here an increasing number of lawsuits are being filed by persons who contract herpes.

To date, the number of cases brought is less than a dozen, and no precedents have been set yet. The appellate process being what it is (or, as you will, what it is not), a final determination may be years away. (Perhaps by then, an available cure for herpes will have been found. At any rate, the irony of such a prospect is irresistible.) The grounds upon which these various cases have been brought are fraud and negligence.

Both presume the defendant to have known he or she had herpes at the time the plaintiff was infected. Negligence is asserted to exist when a person with herpes fails to tell the prospective partner of the disease. In other words, it is asserted the individual has the legal responsibility to notify the partner. Fraud is asserted to exist when a person who knows he or she has herpes is asked whether he or she has herpes and then replies in the negative; i.e., the person lies about not having the disease. Between failure to disclose (negligence) and concealment or misrepresentation (fraud) there is considerable overlap. Furthermore, the vast majority of cases, perhaps, involves the innocent or unwitting transmission of the disease through ignorance despite attempts to prevent it — all without malice. How do these intellectually innocent purveyors of herpes fit into the scheme of things?

Of course, if you want ten different legal opinions on such cases, simply ask ten different lawyers. If you want 20 different legal opinions, first consult ten different lawyers, telling them you are *being sued;* then, have a friend consult those same ten lawyers, telling them to *bring suit.* As is the rule rather than the exception when dealing in matters of law, the validity and legitimacy of such suits are very complicated and have numerous ramifications.

One aspect of these herpes lawsuits, however, is completely uncomplicated and has but one ramification. That single aspect is the fact these herpes lawsuits exist. And, like herpes itself, litigation is a highly contagious and not very selective illness. While perhaps not the most honored tradition in civil law, the notion that "honesty is the best policy" still seems to apply fairly well in the process of conducting one's personal life.

No one wants to get herpes. By the same token, no one should want to pass it on, either. Whether these considerations are genuinely matters for the courts to decide are anybody's guess.

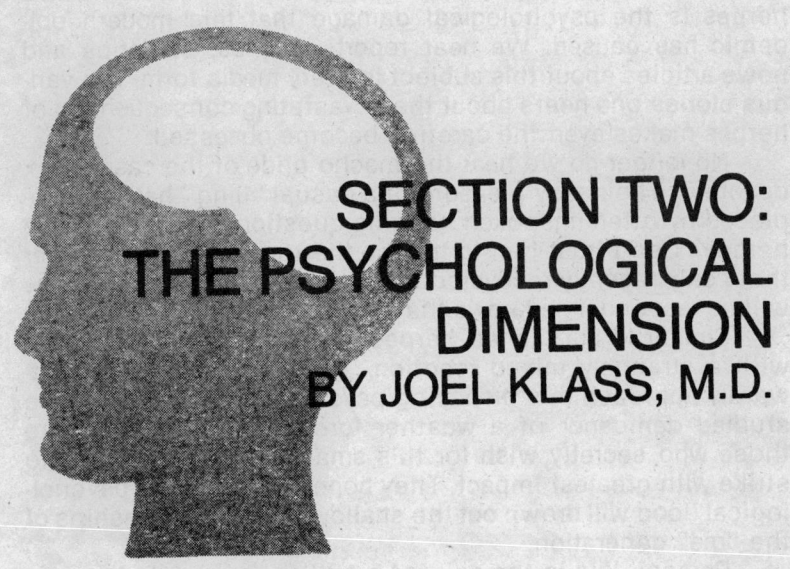

SECTION TWO: THE PSYCHOLOGICAL DIMENSION
BY JOEL KLASS, M.D.

The Destructive Impact

Not since the Black Plague has such a small particle affected the psychology of so many people. The herpes virus threatens to destroy the sexual comfort of an entire nation. From the nagging worry of contracting the bothersome genital lesion of herpes, to the morbid fear that herpes is a precursor of cervical cancer, the sexually active are becoming phobic as never before. Of greater impact than the reports that ten percent of our populaton or 20 million people have contracted herpes is the psychological damage that this modern epidemic has caused. We hear reports, stories, statistics and news articles about this subject in every media form. The various stories one hears about the devastating consequences of herpes makes even the carefree become obsessed.

No longer do we hear the macho pride of the casual sex devotees. Their easy pleasure of a casual "fling" has been replaced by often unspoken nagging questions. Does she have herpes? Can I trust him to tell me the truth? Should I tell her that I only recently recovered from an episode of herpes? How will he respond if he knows that I have had herpes in the past?

Similar to hurricanes, herpes has been met by the public with a strangely mixed reaction. There are those who outwardly approach this menacing psychological storm with the studied demeanor of a weather forecaster. Then there are those who secretly wish for this smallest of viral entities to strike with greatest impact. They hope the damaging psychological flood will drown out the shallow sexual relationships of the "me" generation.

Perhaps this is the guilt of a still Puritan-tainted people who now view herpes as punishment. All too often herpes is viewed as the psychological prison sentence of an all-too-quickly liberated public.

Religionists rejoice in ascribing this epidemic of herpes to the carnal sins of the unrepentant. A new cudgel is swung by fundamentalists to berate the sinful. They proclaim that those who live for sex shall be cursed by sex. They warn that herpes comes as a delayed messenger to call on those who indulge in promiscuous carnal acts.

Has herpes become the answered prayers of the moral majority? Can this so small and dependent particle of life cause such a change in an entire country? Evidently so. The psychological damage is becoming noticeably more evident than the physical trauma. But the full influence of herpes is yet to be seen.

The missionaries of Puritan consciousness are promoting that what the pill can propose herpes may close. They delight that herpes may do more for birth control than the pill ever could. That syphilis used to be seen as a dreaded venereal disease, and is now looked upon as being preferable to herpes, gives substance to their claims.

We are being told that only the beginning is being seen. It is anticipated that this tiny viral spec will become the grain of sand in the shoes of our sexual travelers. The psychological impact of herpes is spreading to infect our nation's minds. It will reside in our thoughts at both the conscious and unconscious level. The psychological impact already reaches the gamut of human emotions: from the bereaved mother who finds her child still-born from herpes' lethal touch to the co-ed's concern about her new date.

The Democracy of Herpes

Whereas before the sexual threat of becoming pregnant was one-sided for women ("she who indulges — bulges") the gender-liberated herpes promises new equality between the sexes. Herpes tags both male and female game players alike. The feeling of being a victim stigmatized by a scar of herpes is no less in the male than the female. Both genders can now as equals see themselves as sexually devalued if they so unwisely choose. Doubts about sexual prowess and self-worth are no longer characteristic of the adolescent. Young and older adults alike suddenly see themselves as less attractive outcasts in their sexual lives when they contract herpes. Herpes serves as an opportunity for anyone to see him or herself as unclean, undesirable and unworthy.

Herpes is often associated with sexual frequency with numerous partners. Many herpes sufferers begin to view themselves as being sexually crippled, psychologically traumatized, and socially devastated.

Digging Into Our Psycho-Social History

The decade of the '50s is often described as that of sexual repression. The '60s, we can easily call the decade of the sexual revolution and the '70s of the pleasure principle and the "me" generation. How then might we describe the '80s?

Certainly venereal awareness or wariness is a likely candidate for an appropriate social description for the decade of the '80s. Even *Time Magazine* gave recognition to the current "harping on herpes" and placed the story in the behavior section of the magazine rather than the medical section, further indicating the greater psychological than physical impact of herpes.

We view our current life style as emphasizing the new American goals. We aspire to psychological and physical health and wealth, uninhibited pleasure and conspicuous consumption. Suddenly herpes threatens to erode the confidence of this age of narcissism. What was a temporary concern about treatable gonorrhea and even syphilis is now a continuing fear about incurable herpes.

The untreatable and unpredictable herpes as well as the potentially devastating mental effect of the herpes plague has its psychological equivalent in *the bomb.* The psychological explosion of herpes has its destructive counterpart in the ever growing concern about the possibility of nuclear war. Both apprehensions prey on the psyche as an ever possible and feebly controlled attack. Whether global or genital, neither leaves us free to view the future without concern. As nations accuse each other of a lack of adequate checks against nuclear proliferation so now individuals all suspect each other of doing irreparable damage because of inadequate herpes precautions. Trust is again developing a meaning for preservation of life and health.

The Denial, the Disgust, the Despair

Sexual deception now has a new indicator test. Infidelity has a new penalty and a new cause is added to the case for virginity and fidelity.

It is becoming evident to many sex therapists that there are those who attempt to deny the effects of the new herpes.

All too often, the result is sexual impotence. Sexual problems also result from an added reason for self-consciousness and worry. Impotence may also result because of the anger upon discovering a history of herpes infection in one's sexual partner. The resulting lack of sexual potency has taken its toll on the sexually active.

Questions about morality arise. Should one freely relate information about his or her state of herpes infection? Is it immoral to transmit the infection without warning? Most individuals have agreed that to not give at least caution is unfair. Having to be wary or even mistrustful has certainly affected the nature of what used to be casual sexual relationships. The one night stand is now followed by the more than one night's insomnia about possible consequences of contracting herpes.

The outbreaks and recurrences of herpes have become a barometer for one's anxiety level. As it is often felt that recurrences are precipitated or aggravated by tension and anxiety the episodes of herpes are now seen as indicators of anxiety level. It is as if a negative biofeedback device has naturally evolved to curtail the sexual life of the promiscuous.

Psychiatrists and psychologists are seeing increasing numbers of depressions relating to herpes. Reactions of anger and even homicidal fantasies are often directed by herpes sufferers towards the donor of their disorder. It may also be directed toward the doctor who cannot cure the disorder or to oneself for "stupidly" contracting the disease. Herpes, with each outbreak, forcibly reminds "the victim" of the original shock of initially discovering the infection. Often heard in the therapist's office is the quote: "I have not seen her for three years but I still get feelings of inner rage every time I think of her and what she gave me". Urologists, internists and gynecologists are seeing increased cases of hypochondriasis relating to herpes. Patients worry that any genital lesion may be the dreaded virus. Concerns about cancer have increased even though with routine health care there are more reported cures than ever before.

Gynecologists are doing more counseling for the concerned pregnant woman who has fears that a previous infection of herpes may become genitally active in time to mortally affect the fetus during delivery. Psychiatrist and psychoanalysts are finding patients focusing on herpes as a just punishment for oedipal (forbidden) desires. Obviously concerns about risking a sexual contact are increasing as never before.

The Disorganized, to the Despondent, to the Demented

Statistically, herpes hits adolescents and young adults more often than other age groups. Although not limited to this age group, herpes is more frequent during this transition to psycho-sexual adulthood. Unfortunately, the psychological toll may be greatest in this period of development, particularly because of a lack of experience and inability in maintaining a proper perspective.

The consequences of discovering a herpes infection and reactions to this discovery are any or all of the following and tend to be in this order:

1. shock, dismay or denial;
2. fear, worry and anxiety;
3. panic and attacks of intense anxiety;
4. anger, regret and helplessness;
5. embarassment, unworthiness and shame;
6. depression and self-hatred;
7. feelings of foreboding, being stigmatized, tainted and stained; and
8. isolation, loneliness, seclusion and social withdrawal.

The initial reaction of shock is generally related to the degree of psychological health and sophistication in the person affected. Generally, the greater the degree of education, maturity, social support and judgment, the less devastating the effects of the discovery of herpes infection.

Anger and helplessness vary depending on the degree of influence the person feels that herpes will have over their life and their future. In addition, premorbid personality structure and ego strengths are most important to preserve good psychological health and diminish the reactions of anger and hopelessness. Feelings of unworthiness and shame are often directly related to the amount of Puritanism in the family of origin of the patient. The greater the intensity of prohibitions the greater the resulting feelings of shame and worthlessness. Often these are the outcome of a fruitless search for a cure and the feeling that the illness being untreatable is the same as terminal. The patient is prone towards all sorts of fads and frauds and feeling even more helpless when these prove useless. Depression sets in as the patient discovers that no amount of effort, medical expertise, money or research can cure them of the disorder. The person begins to retreat from sexual intimacy and social contacts. They fear that their future health, relationships, sexual life and that even children may be denied them.

The view of themselves as bearing a scarlet letter "H" is all too prevalent. They feel the shame stemming from the infection under their belt as publicly disgraceful as if they would wear the proverbial scarlet letter "A" outwardly.

Psychotherapists are seeing more and more individuals who overidentify themselves with the disorder. The resulting poor self-image and low self-esteem indicates that they view themselves as "a herpetic" or venereal leper rather than an individual who has an occasionally bothersome infection. Healthier people generally view themselves and their condition more realistically. They feel that "I'm a person who has a herpes infection with temporary and minimally bothersome recurrences" and not a denigrated subhuman. The pathological response, however, is to become preoccupied with herpes and its consequences. Such individuals become obsessed with herpes as an allegorical figure such as the devil. They feel despondent as their preoccupation with exaggerated effects of their infection diminishes their interest in healthier aspects of life.

The Disorders

Psychiatric disorders that may result from the psychological impact and sequelae of herpes range from mildly increased anxiety to conversion reaction, obsessive-compulsive neuroses and hysteria, to psychotic depressions, paranoia, and precipitation of schizophrenic reactions. An infection of herpes, through its psychological influence, may activate or reactivate many such forms of psychopathology. Even narcissistic personalities can develop significant depressions and decompensation. These disorders are characterized by superficial feelings of well-being related to being impervious to mortal concerns. These personalities are seriously affected by becoming infected by what they see as a periodic loss of control over their lives. They feel a helplessness which generally they demand of themselves to control. They are no longer above others but rather are even forever affected by others through periodic recurrences of herpes.

Other personality types such as the schizoid character may use a herpes infection to rationalize their poor social life. Their already difficult psychosocial development is further complicated by a readily available excuse to avoid involvement with others. The fearful and timid become withdrawn and seclusive.

The inadequate personality and schizoid character disorders become more entrenched with the ever-present threat of herpes derived from contact of others. Along with these disorders conversion reactions can develop depending on the irrational ideation of the patient. Obsessive compulsive individuals gain added fuel as a focal point for their continual preoccupations with excuses for more effective functioning.

Those prone to schizophrenia or paranoia see the infection as exaggerated in its destructive potential. It readily allows their fantasies to proliferate. These fantasies often focus on the destructive punishing aspect of an untreatable infection that is unpredictable in intensity and frequency. The psychological stresses inherent in transitional stages of life such as the young adult or adolescent experience are further complicated by herpes.

Those who read the March 4, 1982 *Rolling Stone* magazine headline "Terrible Curse of Herpes Twenty Million Americans Have It And Will For The Rest of Their Lives" or the *Readers Di-*

gest story of "Grim New Venereal Disease In Our Midst", or *Time* magazine's (June 30, 1980) "Herpes The New Sexual Leprosy" might have lost proper perspective about herpes. Seeing headlines that herpes infects millions with disease and despair or the *Time* magazine (August 2, 1982) "Herpes" article stating that herpes is "an incurable virus which threatens to undo the sexual revolution", may have provided many with undue concern about their sexual lives.

The widespread press coverage of this viral condition has caused a "herpes phobia". Thus, many people with the disease have magnified its significance and let it become a dominant concern in their life. Often it is not even the reality of the herpes but that it is all too easily used as an excuse to avoid areas of already tenuous functioning. They focus their efforts and concern on the physical illness exclusively and thereby avoid the most important psychological ramifications. The example is the patient who obsesses over questions about herpes infections, about its virulence, different forms, recurrences or various body locations rather than accepting valid advice as to how to handle the disorder. These are actually not phobias but exaggerated fears that are promoted by the individual with an unhealthy perspective or personality development. There are even those who do not have herpes but manifest a delusional herpes. That is, they imagine that they have a genital lesion from any unrealistic source and use this to avoid areas of fears. Of course, in these circumstances, treatment of the supposed herpes, even if it were available, would be ineffective. Rather, the real roots of the emotional problem must be uncovered and resolved.

The Dilemma

The whole subject of herpes is strongly colored by the primary concern of those infected. Should a potential lover be informed? How should it be done? Should I take the risk? Shall I trust? What about seeing a psychologist or psychiatrist for my concerns? Should I give in to the base biological urge to continue a sexual impulse or rather give thought to the motivation, my values and my sexual partner?

The Disputes

Of notable concern to marriage counselors and family therapists are the number of patients who focus on herpes as a destructive influence in their relationships. Engagements have been broken, marriages destroyed and sexual lives devastated by irrational concerns over herpes. Much misinformation exists and this gives rise to heated debates between lovers, spouses and even medical practitioners mainly due to misinformation and exaggerations.

Discussions — Case Histories

CASE HISTORY NUMBER ONE

Bert is a 50-year-old married professional who maintains a tenuous second marriage to his much younger wife, Mary, age 32. She has often suspected her husband of infidelity. Bert's infrequent brief affairs have been more to bolster his flagging feelings of masculinity and advancing age than to disparage his spouse.

Mary, without having to confront her husband with incontrovertible evidence, has been able to maintain her denial about his occasional extra-marital affairs. The marriage has been barely satisfactory but sporadically happy.

Bert contracts herpes from a one night stand on a business trip and this experience upsets the precarious marital balance.

Mary reacts more violently than if she had contracted the previous number one sexually transmitted disease, gonorrhea. Although she may be able to deny a single episode she cannot dismiss the recurring attacks of herpes. Each subsequent episode of herpes recalls her original experience of rage. She is unpredictably reinflicted with painful reminders and cannot tolerate this continuing stress. She chooses to divorce.

CASE HISTORY NUMBER TWO

Gil is a pudgy and puerile looking 28-year-old who has never emotionally matured. Although intelligent, his inner insecurities have promoted his relationship to his girlfriend Maggie, an unintelligent and unattractive woman. Frequently boasting of his professional endeavors, Gil has privately felt apprehensive about commencing his sexual life. With embarrassment he relates to Maggie that he is still a virgin. Maggie, recognizing Gil's passivity, nonetheless feels more secure in the fact that she sees him as a safe sexual object. Although not very sexually experienced herself, she has developed a greater comfort than has Gil because of her previous sexual experiences and more confident social life. She pursues Gil and eventually encourages a sexual initiation.

Unfortunately, Gil developes the tell-tale lesions of herpes. After consultation with a physican who matter-of-factly relates the "incurability" of the herpes venereal disease, Gil becomes enraged and severs the relationship with Maggie. He withdraws gradually into an ever more seclusive life style with a paucity of social relationships.

Gil's family notices his increasing depression and withdrawal from life and encourages him to seek professional assistance. His doctor focuses more on giving him a prescription for the disease entity of herpes rather than responding to the more significant psychological effects. Gil is quickly given a prescription for an anti-depressant medication by his physician and dismissed. Gil continues to be despondent and withdrawn with little benefit from medication which is not sufficient to resolve his psychological problems.

CASE HISTORY NUMBER THREE

Marilyn is a 20-year-old college sophomore who comes from an upwardly-mobile highly educated family. She prides herself on establishing meaningful relationships rather than a promiscuous sexual life style. Much to her dismay, however, one such newly-commenced relationship results in her developing genital herpes. She develops an increasing embarrassment and shame as she starts to view herself in disparaging terms. No longer does she feel herself to be a worthy partner of a valued available man but rather a sexual inferior. In her mind she has become one of those that formerly she denigrated as being promiscuous and venereally diseased tramps. Her ensuing poor self-esteem manifests itself in diminishing academic grades as well as an inferior social life. She resorts to a don't-give-a-damn attitude and begins to date only those men she views as safe — those with whom she can feel no shame because of their relatively inferior social status. As she becomes increasingly morose and despondent about an anticipated visit home, and struggling with the pangs of conscience and having to share what she feels she must about her new condition, she takes numerous barbiturate pills, drinks excessively and attempts suicide.

CASE HISTORY NUMBER FOUR

Neil is a neurotic architectural student who tends to blame others for his difficulties, is generally neat but unproductive because of endless hours spent in organizing and reorganizing his work. He shows little relatedness to his emotional awareness. Following his contracting herpes, Neil becomes obsessed with cleanliness. He finds the "incurability" of this infection intolerable and although he intellectually knows this is to no avail he begins handwashing rituals 20 to 30 times daily. He is unable to concentrate on his work because of continual preoccupations with being infested with the contaminating herpes virus. He focuses on his infection as a reason to avoid more meaningful social contacts and eventually gives up on his architectural training because of poor grades. Most unsettling, Neil recognizes increasing rage towards his girlfriend Jane. He questions her continually about the "illicit contact" in which she first acquired the herpes infection and continually berates her for her evil act. He becomes verbally and physically abusive to punish her for damaging his "clean" body and infecting him with an incurable illness.

Neil goes through a succession of relationships, each one destroyed by his continual and unresolved rage about his infection with herpes.

CASE HISTORY NUMBER FIVE

Karen is a 20-year-old clerk in a department store who has had an active dating life but is becoming concerned about the herpes epidemic. She has given little serious thought to her relationships but has rather enjoyed both the social and sexual aspect of her numerous boyfriends.

Karen begins to change her attitudes due to her concern with herpes. She worries about how her boyfriends would react if she contracted herpes and begins to evaluate her last relationships. Although she had been more attracted to men she finds physically attractive, for the first time she realizes that Ken was actually more enjoyable to be with. For the first time, she thinks that an exclusive relationship with him may be more satisfying. Furthermore, she states: "Why take the chance on herpes and how it will affect my life if I should develop it through my casual sexual contacts?"

Karen matures in her judgment and develops a more meaningful relationship with her boyfriend. Her new relationship is based on more lasting qualities and preferences.

CASE HISTORY NUMBER SIX

Michael and Bonnie have been married for three years, have one healthy child and a relatively good marriage. Bonnie has known that Michael had herpes and both have been aware of the available facts about the virus. Whenever Michael has an active lesion and for a short time thereafter, sexual intercourse is avoided. Although Bonnie has voiced concern about contracting the irritating lesion, she recognizes that it is not devastating nor incapacitating. Michael, on the other hand, begins to realize that he is able to delay gratification and need not have immediate sexual satisfaction as he once demanded. Because of this concern about his wife, he is able to abstain from intercourse during those few times he has active lesions. Bonnie, on the other hand, has come to recognize a change in her value system. As she recognizes that she lives in an age in which divorce is all-too-frequent, she begins to place a lower priority on the importance of any inconvenience or irritation she may develop from contracting Michael's herpes. She sees the more intimate and meaningful aspects of the relationship far outweighing these concerns. Surprisingly, both discuss and recognize that they have benefited from the insights they developed in discussing Michael's herpes.

Doctors

As newer and more effective medical treatments are obtained, physicians will apply them. Perhaps of greatest concern, then, is the less than fully available emotional treatment for those affected by herpes.

The following are important approaches to the emotional treatment of herpes:
1. education with accurate information about the infection;

2. support groups and individual medical support emphasizing emotional treatment;
3. individual and group psychotherapies;
4. relaxation techniques and minor tranquilizers;
5. maintaining an atmosphere to allow comfortable ventilation of emotional distress, understanding of individual concerns, and time for these to occur; and
6. more intensive psychotherapy if needed and a reminder that with every adversity there is often an advantage.

Education involves providing up-to-date available sources of information to inform the public and individual patient about readily available treatments as they are developed. In addition, palliative measures can often be taken and certainly psychological resources are available.

Individual and group therapies allow opportunities for ventilation, sharing of feelings and concerns. Patients no longer feel that they are alone and isolated in the manner that someone used to be considered who had leprosy. Social support allows for dissemination of information and sharing of psychological comfort.

Relaxation techniques are particularly effective in decreasing the stress which is thought to often relate to recurrences or to even abort an attack even when prodromal symptoms appear. This may also be true of hypnotic suggestion and self-hypnosis has been proven effective in some for ameliorating or preventing recurrences.

An understanding physician or psychotherapist is invaluable in providing the emotional comfort and opportunity to express individual concerns. This may be sufficient to lessen the stress the individual feels and thereby prevent recurrences of herpes episodes.

Minor tranquilizers such as Ativan, Centrax, Librium, Serax, Tranxene, Valium, Vistaril and Xanax can do much to lessen anxiety in those acutely distressed at the first discovery of having herpes. It may also be effective in lessening the distress of those who are experiencing the burning and itching of a herpes outbreak. This may diminish the length or intensity of the recurring episode. It is important for the individual to maintain a perspective and to see that he or she is a healthy complete individual who has an occasional and limited infection.

It is also important to recognize that benefits may be derived from having herpes: development of better self control in delaying gratification (while waiting for the healing of lesions) before engaging in sexual intercourse as well as more serious assessment of motivations for sexual relations, individual values, and their sexual partners.

Individual psychotherapy offers sufferers of herpes a supportive and beneficial environment. The stress from herpes responds well to short term psychotherapy and to group psychotherapy. The goal of such therapy is not related to herpes but rather the manner in which the individual interprets having herpes.

These psychotherapies may be successfully done by social workers, psychologists, psychiatrists and psychoanalysts. For those who generally need to work on social relationships and do not require medication, working with social workers may be sufficient. If more sophisticated psychological awareness is needed, working with a psychologist may prove profitable. Should the use of medications be indicated or more serious psychiatric disturbances be a possibility, then it is essential that the individual patient seek psychiatric help. This is best done by seeking out a board-certified psychiatrist, that is, a physician with an M.D. degree, who specializes in emotional disorders. Lastly, for complex intrapsychic problems on an unconscious basis it would be advisable to seek the expertise of a psychoanalyst, a physician who specializes in understanding unconscious processes and dreams.

Two frequent levels of psychotherapy are crisis intervention, aimed at ameliorating the immediate severely incapacitating or frightening experience, versus ongoing psychotherapy, which is more appropriate once the crisis stage of panic has subsided. The key is both in a sympathetic and understanding therapist who has full rapport with the patient. If the patient does not feel a rapport with the therapist or progress is not experienced after a few sessions, a frank discussion should be conducted to decide what a realistic goal for therapy is, or if a consultation and a second opinion is indicated.

Group therapy is best undertaken by more experienced therapists trained in psychology or psychiatry. It is best to avoid very charismatic group therapy leaders as these have been associated with a higher "casualty" rate than those who are more client-centered, conservative and fully professional. In group therapy patients derive the added benefit that they may easily dismiss what one therapist may say but find it more difficult to dismiss what an entire group may say. Group confrontation and support are accumulatively effective and may provide a more comfortable and enduring therapeutic response for the patient.

Hypnosis may be used not only to decrease the frequency of recurrences of herpes but also to relieve specific physical symptoms of an attack. The pain, itching and burning can be controlled by an effective hypnotist. Hypnosis may even abort impending attacks. Self-hypnosis can be developed to relieve anxiety and the fears of a spreading infection. Self-hypnosis is best used to contain precipitated neurotic fears. Any positive approach to enhance emotional well-being is always therapeutic. The goal is to minimize stress both to prevent recurrences and minimize current symptoms.

Psychotherapy in general and even more specifically group psychotherapy can be of help to resolve the social concerns and moral issues involved with herpes. What to tell a prospective sexual partner, how to deal with a spouse who develops herpes, and what questions to ask in one's dating life are all important issues that may be addressed through group therapy.

Any physician who is sensitive and understanding to a patient's needs can be effective in helping a patient contend with herpes. Close friends and family members, if the level of communication is sufficiently intimate to allow such discussion, may also be of help. Psychological improvement in any way will improve both the resistance to genital herpes and the adaptation to the disease. Hippocrates long ago stated: "It is more important to know what kind of person has the disease than what kind of disease the person has".

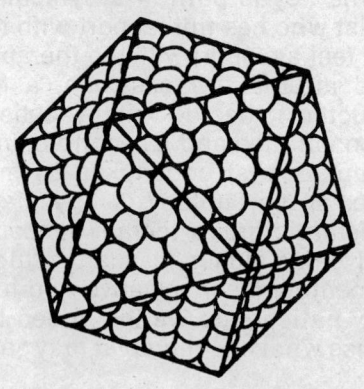

Dialogue

The subject of herpes should be dealt with openly and honestly early in a relationship. If one or the other partner has the virus they should inform the other. Although it is not possible to be 100% sure of not giving it to a partner, every effort can be made to be cautious, refraining from sexual contacts during the times the lesion is active, never knowingly putting a partner at risk.

Much as women carried the burden for centuries of risk in becoming pregnant when they may have chosen not to, today the concern about herpes is more equitable, in which each partner may carry a risk of developing the viral infection.

One need not foment the all too prevalent distortions about herpes. To avoid this, never use the word incurable, terminal or pass on "horror stories" about herpes.

To deal with herpes emotionally, it is important to understand that for practical purposes herpes is *very curable:* the body repeatedly cures reoccurrences at the genital level, and herpes is experienced as only brief intermittent episodes which are increasingly less severe and less frequent. Thus, the best way to think of herpes is as an intermittent, limited condition that is without danger if thoughtfully managed, and which tends to become less bothersome and less frequent with time. Herpes may be forever physically, but it need not be forever emotionally.

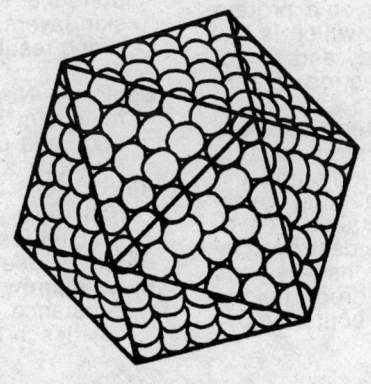

Glossary

Active Immunity — Immunity acquired from prior exposure to an antigen.

Acyclovir — The first antiviral drug licensed by the Food and Drug Administration for manufacture and use in the United States. It is made by Burroughs Welcome Company.

AIDS — Acquired Immune Deficiency Syndrome.

Amniocentisis — Withdrawal of amniotic fluid for examination.

Amniotic Fluid — The fluid in which the fetus is suspended.

Antibiotic — A substance produced either by bacteria, by fungi or is synthesized, which has the ability to inhibit the growth of or kill certain infectious organisms.

Antibody — A type of protein manufactured by certain white blood cells of the lymphatic system in response to an antigen stimulus. Antibodies combine with specific antigens or toxins and render them harmless.

Anus — The lower opening of the digestive tract.

Antigen — A substance, usually protein or a protein sugar complex, which is foreign to the body and stimulates the production of antibodies.

Antiviral — The term supplied to drugs and agents capable of destroying, inhibiting the growth of or inhibiting the development of a virus. The virus then can be destroyed by the body's defense system. Most antiviral drugs belong to the antimetabolite family.

Antimetabolite — A chemical substance similar to a (different) substance required for biological functioning. The antimetabolite serves as a substitute for and interferes with the cellular or viral use of the other, required substance.

Aphthous Stomatitis — A severe infection of small, painful ulcerations — called canker sores — within the mouth. Its cause is unknown, and it often is confused with labial herpes.

Asymptomatic — Without symptoms.

Asymptomatic Carriers — Individuals who harbor disease-causing substances, who transmit disease but who do not manifest disease.

Bag-of-Waters — The uterine sac, filled with amniotic fluid.

Bacteria — Unicellular vegetable micro-organisms, invisible to the naked eye, yet visible under an ordinary optic microscope. Many species cause disease. (Bacteria is plural; bacterium is singular.)

Bleb — A large vesicle or blister, containing fluid. Localized fluid collection beneath the skin causes elevation and separation of the skin layers. Subsequent rupturing results in ulcer formation.

Benign — Non-cancerous, non-malignant or favoring recovery. Used primarily when referring to a tumor.

Birth Canal — The vagina. The path the newborn follows from uterus to outside world.

Blister — See "Bleb".

Bone Marrow — The vascular substance which fills the cavities in the bones.

Canker Sore — See **"Aphthous Stomatitis"**.

Capsid — The protein covering of a virus. It protects the viral DNA.

Carcinogenic — Microscopic protoplasmic masses, surrounded by semi-permeable membranes. A cell is divided into two parts: the nucleus and cytoplasm. They are the fundamental units of life and react biologically with other cells, resulting in the life process.

CDC — Centers for Disease Control, a federal health agency in Atlanta, Georgia, specializing in infectious diseases and epidemiology.

Cell-Mediated Immunity — A type of acquired immunity. It results from the actions of white blood cells manufactured in the thymus gland.

Caesarean Section — Delivery of an infant via incision in the uterine wall, permitting the infant's egress. Though a major surgical procedure, Caesarean sections today are performed routinely.

Cervix — The lower portion, or neck, of the womb. The cervix is located in the upper portion of the vagina, and is a common site of cancer in females.

Chancre — The sore resulting from the initial infection of syphilis.

Chickenpox — A viral disease caused by one of the five members of the herpes family, the varicella-zoster virus. Highly contagious, chickenpox is usually contracted in childhood.

Chromosome — Cellular DNA containing the genes. (See also **"Gene"**.)

Clitoris — The sensitive stimulatory sexual organ of the female, located just anterior to the vaginal opening. Homologue of the male penis.

Conjunctivitis — Inflammation of the mucous membrane lining the inner surface of the eyelids and the anterior portion of the eyes.

Convulsions — Violent involuntary contractions of muscles. A convultions may be generalized or localized. In either case, it results from an abnormal stimulation of nervous system.

Cold Sore — Also called a fever or sun blister.

Cortisone — A steroid hormone secreted by the cortex portion of the adrenal glands.

Cornea — A transparent membrane forming the anterior, or outer, one-sixth of the outer coat of the eyeball. The cornea covers the pupil and lens.

Culture — The propagation of micro-organisms or viruses on or in natural or artificial kinds of media. Usually applied to the growth in a laboratory of bacteria or viruses on tissue specimens or culture media.

Cystitis — An infection of the urinary tract, an inflammation of the bladder.

Cytomegalovirus (CMV) — A member of the herpes virus group. Known to cause a type of pneumonia in those with immuno-deficiency. Often found in association with Kaposi's sarcoma.

Cytoplasm — The contents of a cell, exclusive of the nucleus.

Debilitating Disease — A disease which saps one's strength, causes weakness and malaise.

DNA — Deoxynibonucleic acid, a complex substance of protein and sugar, containing the genetic information of a cell or organism; also the core substance of certain viruses.

Dormant — In a state of suspended physiological activity; in effect, asleep.

Double-Blind Study — Used to determine the effectiveness of a new drug in research studies. Neither the subjects nor the researchers know which subjects are receiving pharmacological agent and which are receiving a placebo.

Drying Agent — A medication, applied topically, that promotes healing by causing a drying effect. Drying agents also help decrease the possibility of secondary infections.

Dye-Light Therapy — An ineffective and dangerous therapy. It formerly enjoyed popularity in the treatment of genital herpes.

Eczema — A skin disorder characterized by local patches of dryness and inflammation, often accompanied by itching, burning or other abnormal sensations in the skin.

Encephalitis — Inflammation of the brain itself. Frequently caused by viruses, but also can be a result of chemical, bacterial, allergic or even non-specific reaction.

Enzyme — Organic substances secreted by living cells. They facilitate biochemical reactions in other substances, though they themselves remain unchanged in the process.

Epidermis — The outermost layer of the skin, and the largest organ of the body.

Epstein-Barr Virus (EBV) — One of the five members of the human being — affecting herpes group. EBV is the causative agent of Infectious Mononucleosis, also called "mono" or the "kissing disease".

Esophagus — The tube, lined with mucous membranes, extending from the back of the throat to the stomach.

Extragenital — Located beyond the genital area.

Exudate — The serum that a lesion exudes.

FDA — The Food and Drug Administration, an agency of the federal government.

Fever Blister — A common descriptive term for a herpes labialis lesion.

Fourchette — The area, in a female, betwen the rectum and the vagina.

Ganglion — Nerve cell bodies-clustered together, external but in close proximity to the brain and spinal cord. Nerve fibers run to and from the ganglion as the fibers course from the brain to the sites within or on the body, and vice versa. (Ganglion is singular; ganglia is plural.)

Gene — An element of DNA containing hereditary information. DNA is composed of multiple genes.

Genetics — The branch of biology dealing with heredity.

Genital — Of or related to a sexual organ.

Gonorrhea — A sexually transmitted disease caused by bacteria called Neisseria gonorrhea. In incidence in the United States, it is second only to herpes simplex.

Gynecologist — A physician who specializes in the treatment of diseases to which only females are subject.

Hepatitis — Inflammation of the liver. Among the causes of hepatitis are viruses, parasitic organisms and toxic chemicals.

Herpes Progenitalis — Medical name for herpes of the genital area.

Herpes Simplex (Type 1 and Type 2) — Two of the five members of the herpes virus family which attack humans. Both types cause labial and genital infections.

Herpes Zoster — Also called the **Varicella-Zoster** herpes virus. The virus which causes chickenpox in children and shingles in adults. Like herpes simplex, herpes zoster can recur. It causes pain along the site of infection's nerve route.

Herpesviruses or **Herpes Viruses** — The viral family, five of whose members can cause infestation in humans. Those five are Herpes Simplex Type 1, Herpes Simplex Type-2, Varicella-Zoster, Epstein-Barr and Cytomegalovirus.

Hormones — Substances secreted by glands and which circulate in the bloodstream, affecting cells in other parts of the body.

Host — Any organism or cell invaded by a parasite. For example, humans are the natural hosts of the herpes simplex viruses. Human skin and mucous membrane cells are the usual host cells of herpes viral invasion.

Humoral Immunity — The portion of the immune system responsible for producing circulating antibodies. Antibodies fence off producing circulation antibodies. Antibodies fend off bacterial or viral invasion or neutralize foreign, toxic substances.

Hypersensitivity — An exaggerated response to a foreign stimulus.

Hysterectomy — The surgical removal of the uterus, or womb. The ancidents believed the removal of this organ caused hysteria, thus the Greek word hysteros was applied to the organ.

Immune — Unsusceptible; capable of mounting a defense adequate to resist the invasion of an offending agent.

Immune Response — The collective efforts of the body's defensive system when fighting a disease or chemical toxin.

Immune System — The physiological and bio-chemical resources of the body to defend itself against foreign invasion.

Immunocompromised — The weakening of the immune defense system of the body, leaving the body unable to mount a successful white blood cell or antibody response to invasion. Most often the result of chemotherapy or of a chronic debilitating disease.

Immunodeficient — An immune defense system that fights infections or toxins inefficiently.

Immunize — The process of making an organism immune to a specific antigen.

Infection — As applied to viral illness, the invasion of an establishment of a stronghold in the body by the virus.

Initial Infection — As applied to viruses, the first clinical infection in the host organism of the specific virus in the presence of antibodies to to the herpes virus in the blood. Initial outbreaks usually are less severe than primary infections because the immune system of the host has had prior contact with the virus.

Interferon Inducers — Substances which stimulate host cells to secrete interferon.

Iris — The colored portion of the eyeball. The iris surrounds the pupil.

Kaposi's Sarcoma — Malignant tumors of skin and mucous membrane associated with AIDS.

Keratitis — Inflammation of the cornea of the eye. Often caused by the herpes virus.

Labia — The word means lips. It commonly is used to refer to the labial lips of the vagina. The term herpes labialis, however, is used to designate herpes of the lips of the mouth.

Latency — Inactive period of infestation. During a latent period, the virus is dormant (see **"Dormant"**) and not actively producing the disease. The latent herpes virus remains so in the nerve ganglion nearest the site of infestation.

Lesion — Any sore or ulceration. The herpes virus spreads cell-to-cell, and a herpes simplex lesion appears when and where the virus has attacked and destroyed many cells within a small, specific area. Characteristically, the herpes simplex lesion is a blister resembling a chickenpox lesion.

Lumbo-Sacral Ganglion — The nerve root at the base of the spine which supplies nerve fibers to the genital area. The lumbo-sacral ganglion is the common site of the dormant herpes virus involved in a genital infection.

Lymph Gland or **Node** — An anatomical accumulation of lymphoid tissue. A lymph node produces and stores lymphocytes.

Lymphocytes — White blood cells which are the basis of the cellular immune defense system. Lymphocytes attack and destroy antigens.

Lysine — An essential amino acid. This protein component retards the growth of the herpes virus in laboratory cultures, or "in vitro", but has not been shown to be effective "in vivi".

Lysis — The process of cellular disintegration or explosion.

Macrophage — A giant cell which eats other cells and debris. The macrophages are an important component of the cellular immune defense system. Stored in the bone marrow, the macrophages devour antigens and cells invaded by the virus.

Malignant — Resistant to treatment. Tending to grow worse. Used as in a cancer tumor which spreads from original site to other parts of the body.

Meningitis — Infection or inflammation of the membranous tissue which surrounds the brain or spinal cord. Meningitis usually is caused by bacteria, but also can be caused by a virus, a fungus, a chemical or be of diffuse origin from a severe, inflammatory illness.

Mucous — The viscid secretion a cell produces to lubricate and protect its membrane.

Mucous Membrane — The cellular lining of body cavities. These linings secrete mucus. The particular cavity may or may not communicate directly with the body's exterior.

Neonate — Newborn.

Neonatal — Referring to the neonate.

Neoplasm — A new tissue growth; a tumor. A neoplasm serves no useful purpose, and may be benign or malignant.

Nerve Pathways — The neural path a nerve impulse takes from and to its ganglion and ultimately to the brain.

Neuralgia — Pain experienced along a nerve pathway.

Non-Primary Infection — A first infection of herpes at a body site in an individual who has had a previous herpes infection at a different body site. Circulating antibodies offer partial protection against the new viral invader.

Non-Venereal Herpes — Herpes infestation not resulting from any form of sexual activity.

Nucleus — The round inclusion approximately at the center of a cell. The nucleus directs cellular functions and contains the chromosomes and other genetic data.

Nucleic Acid — An acid derived from sugar, phosphoric acid and a base substance. Nucleic acid usually is located within the nucleus of a cell. DNA is one type of a nucleic acid.

Obstetrician — A physician who provides pre-natal care and who assists in the delivery of infants.

Pap Smear — A method of examining tissue to determine the presence or absence of cancerous or pre-cancerous cells. A Pap smear also can detect tissue changes due to the presence of a viral invader. It frequently is used to examine tissue specimens scraped from the cervix. Named after its originator, Dr. George Papanicolau.

Parasite — An organism living on or within, and at the expense of, another (the host) organism.

Passive Immunity — Immunity acquired from the passage of antibodies that formed outside the recipient's body. Compared with active immunity, passive immunity is short-lived.

Phagocytes — Cells that ingest foreign antigens, foreign cells or cellular debris. Part of the cellular immune defense system.

Photoinactivation Therapy — See "Dye-Light Therapy".

Phobia — A persistant, irrational and abnormal fear of an object or of a situation, the object or situation itself having no basis in reality to provoke concern or alarm.

Placenta — The organ affixed to the uterine wall which establishes communications between mother and fetus via the umbilical cord. it serves to supply nutrition to the fetus, transfer antibodies from mother to fetus and remove waste products from the fetus.

Primary Herpes — The first infection of the herpes simplex virus in an individual who never has been infected with either (Type-1 or Type-2) herpes simplex strain. No antibodies against HSU-1 or HSU-2 circulate in the bloodstream.

Placebo — A pharmacologically inert substance used for psychological effect. In controlled drug studies, placebos are used to measure the *imagined* benefits derived from the substance being tested.

Placebo Effect — A benefit or improvement a subject notes and attributes to medication or treatment when no such intrinsic benefit or improvement exists.

Prodrome — Those sensations experienced by an individual prior to the outbreak of herpetic lesions.

Proctitis — Inflmmation of the rectal, anal or peri-anal tissue. Its cause may be either venereal or non-venereal.

Psychiatrist — A physician who specializes in the treatment of emotional or mental disorders.

Psychologist — An individual trained in the science dealing with mental and emotional behavior.

Reactivation — In herpes, the change in status of the virus from dormant to active.

Recurrent Herpes — Virus attack subsequent to an initial one, resulting from the dormant virus travelling along the nerve path and becoming active at the site of original infestation.

Replication — Viral reproduction.

Reportable Disease — A disease the law requires physicians to report to health authorities.

Secondary Infection — An infection superimposed upon an existing infection, caused by a pathogen other than the one causing the existing infection.

Shedding — As applied to herpes, the state of viral infection in which viral particles are present on the surface of the skin or mucous membrane.

Shingles — A condition caused by the herpes-zoster virus.

STD — Acronym for *sexually transmitted disease.* Formerly known as VD, or venereal disease.

Steroid — A complex, chemical-base structure found in cortisone drugs and in hormones.

Subclinical — A disease condition usually not detectable by visual observation.

Syphilis — A contagious venereal disease caused by a member of the bacterial family called Treponema Pallidum.

Target Cells — Cells marked for destruction because antigens enable the body to recognize them as having non-self components.

Trauma — An injury to tissue or to the psyche.

Trigeminal Ganglion — The ganglion of the fifth, or trigeminal, nerve, located near the base of the brain.

Tissue — An aggregate, or collection of cells or of derivatives of cells, forming a definite structure.

Topical — Of or pertaining to the skin or a mucous membrane surface.

Trigger — An event, substance or other factor that initiates a recurrent attack of herpes.

Tumor — A circumscribed growth of tissue, not inflammatory in character and arising from pre-existing tissue. In general use, any swelling of tissue. In limited use, a neoplasm.

Tzanck Smear — A test for viral replication, similar to the pap smear.

Ulcer — A loss of skin or of mucus membrane in a localized area, usually accompanied by irritation and inflammation until it heals.

Urethra — The tubular structure connecting the bladder to the exterior of the body.

Ultraviolte Rays — The rays of the sun which cause harmful effects upon the skin. Ultraviolet rays are beyond the spectrum of visible light.

Vaccination — The inoculation of the body with a non-pathogenic virus or bacterium similar to a related yet pathogenic species. This enables the body to acquire an immunity against the pathogenic species.

Vagina — The tube-like structure extending from the cervix to the exterior of the body in a female, and which serves as the birth canal.

Varicella — Chickenpox.

Venereal Disease — See "STD".

Vesicle — A blister, characterized by a raised segment of skin filled with fluid.

Vesicular Fluid — The fluid contained within a vesicle.

Viricide — A substance capable of killing a virus.

Virus — Obligate parasite which reproduces only in the presence of and in conjunction with living tissue.

Vulva — The female labia majora and the cleft between them.

Whitlow — Herpetic infection of a finger.

White Blood Cell — A type of blood corpuscle, also called a leukocyte. White blood cells originate in the bone marrow.

Zovirax® — The brand name for the drug acyclovir.

Index

A

Abdoomen, 47
Abortion, spontaneous, 63-64
Abrasions, 17-18
  AIDS and, 89
Abstinence, 48, 50, 53, 106
Acquired Immune Deficiency Syndrome (AIDS), 86-92
Acyclovir (ACV), 9, 58
  indiscriminate use of, 59
  intravenous, 38, 41
Adenine arabinoside (Ara-A), 39-40
AIDS, (See Acquired Immune Deficiency Syndrome)
Alcohol solution, 61
Allergic dermatitis, 38
American Social Health Association (ASHA), 85
Amino acids, 56
Amniotic fluid, 67, 69
Amylnitrite, 86
Anal sexual activities, 23, 89
Analgesics, 39
Anger, 99-101
Antibodies, 31, 44-45, 56, 66-67, 72, 80
  in infants, 66
  recurrences and, 31
  viruses and, 77
Antibiotics, 9, 41, 90
Anti-depressants, 105
Antimetabolite drugs, 59
Antiviral drugs, 9, 59
Antiviral research, 9
Anus, 13-14, 23, 64
Anxiety, 99-100, 102, 108, 110
  recurrences and, 52
  relief from, 51
Appetite, loss of, 21, 88
Aqueous solution, 61
Ara-A, 39-40
Ara-C, 40
Ara-AMP, 40
Arginine, 56
Aspirin, 61
Astruc, Jean, 8, 15
Ativan, 108
Atopic dermatitis, 38
Autoinoculation, 18-19

B

Babies (see Infants)
Bacteria, 22, 60
Bacterial infection, 24, 38
Bacterial paronychia, 41
Bateman, Thomas, 15
Bathing, 61
BCG (Bacille Calmette-Guerin), 56
Benson's Relaxation Response, 32
Betadine soap, 55
Biofeedback, 32, 99
Birth, 36, 64-65, 69
Birth control techniques, 83, 97
Birth defects, 65
Bladder, 13, 24, 64
Bleeding, 40
Blindness, 9, 35, 65
Blisters, (See Also Lesions), 21-22, 29-30, 35, 80
  breaking open of, 20, 26
  fever, 26, 70
  in diagnosis of disease, 22
  on the mouth, 42
Blood, 89-90
Blood antibodies, typed, 45
Blood sharing, 90
Bloodstream, 77, 79
Blood tests, 22, 44
Blood transfusion, 91
Body defenses, 73
Boils, 22
Bone marrow, 81
  transplants of, 90
Bowel movements, 21, 23
Brain, the, 28, 38
  infection of, 39
Brain damage, 39
  infant herpes and, 65
Brain herpes, (encephalitis), 9, 12
Bromovinyldeoxyuridine (BVDU), 59
Burkitt's Lymphoma, 88
Burning sensation, 21, 30, 35, 51, 58, 108, 110
  and uric acid, 24
Burroughs Welcome Company, 58
Buttocks, 13, 23, 30, 47

C

Caesarean incision, 64
Caesarean section, 64, 69
Cancer, 71, 86, 100
  and AIDS, 91
  cervical, 46, 72, 96
  dye-light therapy and, 56
  vulvar, 72
Canker sores, 23
Capillary blood vessel, 18
Capsid, 72-73, 76-77
Carbon dioxide laser treatment, 60
Carunculae Hymenales, 14
Cataracts, 37
Cells, 15, 18, 60, 72-73, 80-81
  skin, 31
  tumor, 88
Cell-mediated immunity, 80
Centrax, 108
Centers for Disease Control (CDC), 9
Cervical cancer, 9, 46, 72, 96
Cervical herpes, 72
Cervical infection, 50
Cervix, 13, 21, 26, 36, 46-47, 64, 72
Chancroid, 22
Cheeks,
  canker sores inside of, 23
Chickenpox, 8
  lesions of, 35
Childbirth, 32, 61
Children, oral herpes and, 17, 42
Chills, 25
Chronic cutaneous herpes simplex, 41
Circumcision, 27
Cirrhosis, 40
Clitoris, 13
Clinical study, 20
Clothing, tight, 50
CMV, 86-87
Cold, the common, 15, 76, 84, 86, 88
Cold sores, 8, 15-18, 22, 26
  from fever, 16
  from sunburn, 16
  on lips, 12
  on mouth, 8
Complications, 39
Compresses, cold or ice, 61
Condoms, 47, 84
Congenital herpes, 68
Contact transmission, 17, 19, 48
Contagiousness, 12, 18, 25
  of AIDS, 89-90
Contraceptive gels, 47
Contraceptives, 47
Contracting herpes, 10, 17, 24, 27, 34, 42, 47-50, 53-54, 82-84, 93, 96-97, 99, 104-107
  infants and, 67, 69, 70-71
Control, 47

Coping, 9
Cornea, the, 35
Cortisone, 61
Cowpox, 75
Crawling feelings, 30
Cultures, viral, 24, 43-44, 48, 53, 68-69
Cures, ineffectiveness, 15, 55, 61, 101
Cytomegalovirus (CMV), 86-87
Cytology, 44
Cytologists, 46

D

Defense system, 58, 79-80
Dehydration, 42
Delivery, 65-66, 68-69, 100
  premature birth, 64
Delusional herpes, 103
Dentists, 42
Deoxyribonucleic acid (DNA), 45
Depression, 99-100, 102, 105
Dermatitis, allergic or atopic, 38
Despair, 100, 103
Diagnosis, of herpes, 20, 22-23, 35, 39, 43-44, 46, 54, 60
  of AIDS, 90-91
Diet, 23, 31, 56, 61
Diarrhea, 88
Diaphragms, 18, 47, 84
Digestive tract, 40
Dimethylsulfoxide (DMSO), 55
Disorders, psychiatric, 102
Diuretic, 52
Divorce, 104
DMSO, 55
DNA, 45, 60, 71-73, 76-78
Doctors, 42, 107
  advice of, 10, 42
  anger against, 99
  relationship with, 10
Dormancy, 9, 12, 27-29, 31, 36, 48, 53, 64, 81
Douche, pregnancy and, 63
Drugs, 9, 58-61, 91
  experimental, 38, 46
Drug users, 86, 90
DUNHL, 88
Dye-light therapy, 55-56

E

Eczema, herpes, 38

Electron microscopy, 69
Emotions, 10, 103, 107, 109
Emotional stress, 30
Encephalitis, 9, 12, 39, 91
Epstein-Barr virus, 88
Esophagus, 40
Exercise, 51
Experiments, 34
Eye, herpes and the, 9, 12, 17-18, 28, 35, 37

F

Face, the, 28, 37
Facial herpes, 39
False positive tests, 23
Family therapists, 104
Fatigue, 30, 57, 88
FDA, 58-59
Fear, 100, 103, 110
Fetid breath, 42
Fetus, 67, 100
Fever, 21, 24, 37-38, 42, 61, 88
  cold sores from, 16
  in recurrent attacks, 25
Fever blisters, 26, 70
FIAC, 59
Fibroblast, 59
Fingers, 19, 23, 41
Flu, 84, 88
Fluorescent Treponema Antibody Absorption Test (FTA), 22-23
Folliculitis, 22
Fourchette, 13-14
Foreskin, 13, 27
FTA test, 22

G

Gall bladder, 40
Ganglia, 29
Ganglion, 28
Ganglion cell, 29
Ganglion nerve, 27-29, 31
Gay population, 23
Genital herpes, 17-23, 25-27, 33-34, 40, 45, 48-49, 53, 59, 66, 72, 82-84, 105, 111
  diagnosis of, 46
  pregnancy and, 63-64, 68-69
  primary, 25, 37
  prevalency of, 16
  recurrent, 38, 58, 82
  transmission of, 19
Genitalia, 12, 18, 85
Genital infections, primary, 63

recurrent attacks, 13
Genital tract, 22
Glands, 12
  swollen, 35
Gentian violet, 61
Glaucoma, 37
Gonorrhea, 20, 34, 98, 104
  rectal, 24
Groin, swelling of, 21, 23
Group therapy, 109
Gums, canker sores at base of, 23
Gynecologists, 99-100

H

Hair follicles, 22
Hand, 18-19, 37, 51-52, 70
Head, 12
Headaches, 38
Heat, 34, 61
Heat sensations, 30
Heartburn, 40
Hemophilia, 90
HELP support groups, 85
Helper, The, 85
Helplessness, feelings of, 100-102
Hepatitis, B, 90
Hepatitis, viral, 76
Herpes cervicitis, 64
Herpes eczema, 38
Herpes encephalitis, 39
Herpes meningitis, 38
Herpes phobia, 96, 103
Herpes Resource Center (HELP), 85
Herpes simplex virus, 29, 75
  and AIDS, 88
  cancer and, 71
  contracting, 10, 17
  definition of, 12
  diagnosis of, 22
  epidemic aspects of, 9, 16
  genital, 8, 12
  growth rate, 16
  history of, 15
  homosexuals and, 86
  immune system, 77
  infection, 31, 79
  infidelity and, 104
  initial infection, 66
  legal aspects, 93-94
  life-cycle of, 73, 76, 78
  newborns and, 9, 12
  oral, 12-15, 17
  pregnancy and, 63
  psychological aspects of, 10, 96
  recurrences, 8-9, 12, 15, 30
  resources, 85

121

shape of, 74-75
strains of, 12, 14
symptoms, 9, 19-22, 24-25, 35-38, 40, 44, 48, 61, 68, 70
transmission of, 12
viral spread of, 78-79
typing, 45
Type 1 (HSV-1), 8, 12, 14-15, 18, 20, 26, 28, 35-36, 38-39, 41, 45-46, 58-59, 66, 70
Type 2 (HSV-2), 8, 12, 14, 20, 26, 35-36, 38, 41, 45-46, 58-59, 66, 70
History of herpes epidemiology, 14
Herpes whitlow, 70
Hiatus hernia, 40
Hippocrates, 110
History, medical, 8, 15, 22
Home remedies, 61
Homosexuality, 86, 88, 90, 92
   AIDS and, 86
   sexual promiscuity and, 92
Host cell, 26, 43-44, 46, 59, 73, 76-81
Host organism, 73, 81
Hot tub, 34
Humoral immunity, 80
Hygiene, 34, 37, 49-50, 52, 61, 92
   in AIDS prevention, 92
Hygienists, 42
Hypnosis, 57, 108, 110
Hypochondria, 99
Hysteria, 102

I

Icosahederal, shape, 74-75
Immune system, 26, 29, 31-33, 60, 66-67, 79-81, 87-88
   childrens, 42
   deficient, 41
   immunosuppression, 41, 87
   infants, 66, 71
   newborns and, 65
Immuno-chemical methods, 45
Immunosuppression, 41, 86-88, 90
Immunological system, 31
Impotence, 99
Incubation period, 19
Infants, 70-71, 79-80
   AIDS and, 90
   fatality rate from herpes and, 66-67
Infection, 18, 22, 25, 27, 30-32, 38, 43-44, 48, 52, 60, 70, 79, 81, 86
   AIDS and, 90
   bacterial, 38
   initial, 12, 21, 26, 66
   in utero, 67
   latent, 17
   primary herpes simplex virus and, 13, 19, 22, 26, 33, 36, 66-68
Infectious mononucleosis, 8, 88
Influenza, 75
Interferon, 59-60, 91
Internists, 99
Iris, the, 37
Itching, 21, 30, 51, 108, 110

J

Jogging, 51

K

Kaposi's sarcoma, 86-88, 90-91
Keratin, 18
Keratitis, 35-37
Kissing, 15, 18, 70, 92
   children, and, 70
Knees, 30

L

Labia, 13-14
Labial herpes, 39
Labialis, 70
Laboratory tests, 43
Larynx (vocal cords), 42
Lasers, 60-61
Lasers, surgery with, 15
Legal aspects, 93-94
Lesbianism, 89
Lesions, 12, 17, 20-23, 25, 27, 31-33, 39, 42-44, 47-48, 51, 56-57, 60, 62, 68, 72, 77, 80-81, 105, 107, 111
   cervical, 21
   genital, 15, 19, 23, 34, 37, 42, 61, 65, 96, 99, 103
   on eye, 66
   on mouth, 15, 35, 61, 66
   on skin, 12, 25, 41, 66, 70, 72
   oral, 13
   penile, 29
   psoriatic, 38
   rectal, 21
   urethral, 24
   vaginal, 21
Librium, 108
Lips, 12-13, 18-19, 28, 35-36, 70-71
   cancer of, 35
   canker sores inside of, 23
   cold sores on, 12, 16
Lithium, 11, 56
Liver, the, 90
Living organism, 74
Lymph, 77
Lymph glands, 88
Lymph nodes, 22-23, 35, 42, 81
Lymph tissues, 90
Lymphoma, 88
Lysine, 56-57, 61

M

Macrophages, 81
Malaise, 21, 30
Marrigage, 10, 53, 104, 107
Masturbation, 19
Measles, 76
Media, 82, 87, 96
Meditation, 32
Meningitis, herpes, 38-39
Menstruation, 30, 51
Mental aspects, 49, 84
Milk of Magnesia, 61-62
Mononucleosis, 8, 88
Mortality rate, herpes of the brain, 39
Mouth, the, 12-15, 20, 28, 61, 70-71
   blisters on 15
   canker sores within, 23
   cold sores on, 12
   fungus infection in, 88
   herpes of, 42
Mucous, 90
Mucous membranes, 17, 28-29, 31, 79
Mumps, 76

N

Natural host, 34
Nausea, 38
Neck, the, 35
   stiffness in, 38
   swollen glands of, 37
Neonatal herpes, 9, 65-66, 70
Narcissistic personalities, 102
Nerve cells, 27-28

Nerve centers, 30
Nerve fiber, 27, 29
Nerve ganglion, 27, 30-31
Nervous system, 28, 57
  and diagnosis, 39
Neuralgia, 30
Newborn child, 12, 36, 70-71
  congenital herpes and 68
  diagnosis of, 39, 66
  herpes and 64-65, 69
New England Journal of Medicine, The, 58
Night sweats, 88
Nutritional supplements, 61
Nurses, 42

O

Obsessive-compulsive neuroses, 102, 106
Ocular herpes, 9, 12, 17-18, 28, 35, 37
Ointments, 58
Olfactory nerve, 39
Oral herpes, 12-17, 19-20, 39-40, 58
  sores of, 42

P

Pain, 9, 13, 21, 24-25, 27, 30, 35, 42, 61, 110
  bowel movements and, 23
  of the eye, 37
  on urination, 24
  rectal, 23
Pap smear, 46, 72
  during pregnancy, 69
Papanicolaou, Dr. George, 45
Paranoia, 102
Paronychia, 41-42
Pathologists, 15, 46, 91
Pelvic ache, 21
Pelvis, 37
Penis, 12-13, 50
  recurrent attacks on, 25
Perianal area, 23
  lesions on, 21
Photophobia, 37
Physicians, 10, 22, 82
Pill, the, 83, 97
Pinkeye, 37
"Pins and needles", 30
Placebo effect, 56-57
Placenta, 66-67, 69
Plasma exchange transfusion, 90-91
Pneumonia, 88, 91
Polio, 75-76
Pox virus (small, cow), 75
Premature deliveries, 63
Pregnancy, 9, 43, 66, 68, 83, 97, 100, 111
  first (primary) infection and, 64, 66, 69
Premenstrual tension, 52
Prenatal monitoring, 44
Prevention, 47, 50, 53, 62, 68, 83
Proctitis, 24
Prodromal symptoms, 30-32, 48, 51, 58, 68, 108
Prostate gland, 13
Prostitution, 83
Psoriasis, 38
Psychiatrists, 99-100, 103, 109
Psychoanalysis, 100, 109
Psychological aspects, 32, 96, 98, 100, 102, 105
  delusional herpes, 103
  emotional impact, 10, 97
  trauma, 10
Psychologists, 99, 103, 109
Psychopathology, 102
Psychotherapists, 101, 108
Psychotherapy, 110
  group, 108, 110
  individual, 108-109
Psychotic depressions, 102

R

Rabies, 76
Reactivation (see Recurrent attacks)
Reader's Digest, 102-103
Recipients of blood, 80
Rectum, the, 13, 23-24, 64
  cancers of, 88
  infections of, 24
Recurrent attacks, 12-13, 15, 17, 19, 22-23, 25-27, 29-33, 35, 38-39, 41, 44-45, 47-53, 58, 60-61, 67-68, 70, 81, 99, 103-104, 108
  causes of, 30
  duration of, 31, 55-56, 67, 81, 108, 111
  frequency of, 31, 33, 55, 67, 81, 110-110
  genital, 13
  of urinary tract, 25
  personal effects of, 102
  pregnancy and, 66
  prevention through hypnosis, 110
  severity, 55-56, 67, 81, 108, 111
  sexual activities and, 63
Red blood cells, 74-75
Relationships, 10, 49
Relaxation techniques, 108
Replication, viral, 29, 31, 59-60, 77
Research, 9
Research studies, 40
Respiratory therapists, 42
Rheumatic disorders, 55
Rolling Stone, The, 102
Rome, ancient, 15

S

Sacral ganglion, 28, 38
Saline solution, 61
Saliva, 17-19, 37, 42, 70, 80-90
Scabies, 25
Scab formation, 20
Scabies, 22
Scarring, 21, 97
Schizoid character, 102
Schizophrenic reactions, 102
Scrotum, 47
Self-esteem, 84, 101, 105
Self-inoculation, 37
Self-image, 101
Self-worth, 97
Semen, in spread of disease, 17, 25, 89-90
Sensory ganglion cell, 29
Serax, 108
Serum viral titer test, 43
Sexual activity, 17, 19, 27, 30, 32, 37, 42, 47, 49, 50-54, 83-84, 96-97, 99, 101, 103-106, 109
  avoiding, 47, 63, 111
  between attacks, 33
  changes in, 82
  deception about, 99
  homosexual activity, 87
  oral, 14, 17, 19
  pregnancy during, 63
  reactivation of disease and, 53
  recurrences and, 52
Sex education, in schools, 53-54
Sex therapists, 99
Sexually transmitted disease (STD), 8, 12, 19-20, 42, 50, 54, 85-86, 89, 104
Shame, 101, 105
Shedding of virus, 25, 30, 42, 48, 53, 58, 67-68
Shedding, silent viral, 24, 69-70, 77

Shingles, 8, 35
Sitz baths, 24
Skin, the, 12, 17-18, 27-30, 38, 40, 50, 70, 79-80
   infections of, 40
   lesions on, 12
   minor irritations of, 22
   strange sensations on or beneath, 23
Small pox, 75
Smoking, 51
Snake venom, 55
Social withdrawal, 100, 105
Sociological aspects, 82
Spermicidal jellies, 84
Spermatic cord, 13
Spinal cord ganglion, 28
Spirochetes, 23
Staining test, 35
Statistics, 100
Steroids, 61
Stool softeners, 23
Stress, 32, 51, 104, 108
   emotional, 30
   mental, 51, 81
   minimizing, 110
   physical, 51, 70
   psychological, 102
   recurrent attacks and, 23
Stress management techniques, 32
Sunburn, cold sores from, 16
Sunlight, 51
Sunscreens, 52
Surgery, 91
Support groups, 108
Swallowing, difficulty in, 40
Sweat, 89-90
Swimming pool, 84
Symptoms of herpes, 9, 19-22, 24-25, 30, 35-38, 40, 44, 48, 61, 68, 70, 110
Syphilis, 20, 22-24, 34, 97-98

T

Testicle, 13
Thighs, 13, 47
   pain in, 23
Throat, the, 37
Throbbing, 30
Tiberius, Emperor, 15
Time Magazine, 98, 103
Tincture solution, 61
Tingling, 30, 51, 58
Tissue cells, 43
TM, 32
Toilet seats, 34
Tongue, the, 12
   cancers of, 88
Tonsillitis, 37

Topical treatments, 58-59, 61
Tranquilizers, 108
Transfer factor, 91
Transmission of virus, 18, 34, 36, 46, 50, 63, 82-84
   to newborns, 70
   to other parts of the body, 10
   VD and, 19
Trannxene, 108
Trauma, physical and psychological, 97-98
Treatment, 15, 20, 22, 37-38, 46, 54-56, 60, 82, 107
   breakthroughs in, 15-16
Trench mouth, 35
Trigeminal ganglion, 28, 36, 38-39
Triggers, 53, 70
   stress as, 32, 81
Tuberculosis, 56
Tumors
   associated with AIDS, 88
   on mucous membranes, 86
   on skin, 86
Type 1 Herpes, 8, 12, 14-15, 18, 20, 26, 28, 35-36, 38-39, 41, 45-45, 58-59, 66, 70
Type 2 Herpes, 8, 12, 14, 20, 26, 28, 35-36, 38, 41, 45-46, 58-59, 66, 70

U

Ulcerations, 80
Ulcers, 40-41
   aphthous, 23, 61
   bleeding peptic, 40
   in rectal canal, 23
   of the eyes, 37
Ultraviolet rays, 51-52, 55
Undergarments, 50-51
United States, 9, 27, 36, 88-89
Upper gastrointestinal symptoms, 40
Urethra, 13, 64
   lesions in 24, 29
Urethral channel, 13, 25, 50
Urethral orifice, 14
Uric acid, 24
Urinary retention, 24
Urinating after sex, 50
Urination, 24
   pain with, 21, 24
   difficulty with, 23, 27
Urologists, 99
Uterus, the, 67-68

V

Vaccines, 56, 62
   of the future, 62
Vagina, the, 13, 17, 21, 24, 26, 36, 50-51, 64-65
Valium, 108
VD National Hotline, 85
Venom, snake, 55
Venereal disease (VD), 8, 15, 19, 97, 105
Vesicles, (See Lesions)
Vidarabine (Ara-A), 39, 59
Vira-A, 39
Viremia, 65, 67, 69
Virion, 74
Viruses, 29, 31, 33, 43-44, 46, 48, 50, 67, 76-81, 83, 86-87, 100, 103
   definition of, 73-74
   resistance to, 49
   types of, 33
Virulence, 26, 33, 91, 103
Vistaril, 108
Vitamins, 61
Vitamin E, 55
Vomiting, 38
Vulva, 50
Vulvar cancer, 72

W

Washing, 50-51
White blood cells, 59, 74-75
Whitlows, 41-42
Worry, 100

X

Xanax, 108

Y

Yellow fever, 56
Yoga, 51

Z

Zinc, 61
Zovirax, 58

Imperial Public Library
Imperial, Texas